Medical Humanities Companion

VOLUME TWO

Medical Humanities Companion
VOLUME TWO

Diagnosis

Edited by
Rolf Ahlzén
Martyn Evans
Pekka Louhiala
and
Raimo Puustinen

Series Editors
Rolf Ahlzén, Martyn Evans, Pekka Louhiala
and Raimo Puustinen

Radcliffe Publishing
Oxford • New York

Radcliffe Publishing Ltd
18 Marcham Road
Abingdon
Oxon OX14 1AA
United Kingdom

www.radcliffe-oxford.com

Electronic catalogue and worldwide online ordering facility.

British Library Cataloguing in Publication Data

A catalogue record for this book is available from the British Library.

ISBN-13: 978 184619 464 1

The paper used for the text pages of this book is FSC certified. FSC (The Forest Stewardship Council) is an international network to promote responsible management of the world's forests.

Mixed Sources
Product group from well-managed forests and other controlled sources
www.fsc.org Cert no. SGS-COC-2482
© 1996 Forest Stewardship Council

Typeset by Pindar NZ, Auckland, New Zealand
Printed and bound by TJI Digital, Padstow, Cornwall, UK

Contents

About the series editors

Rolf Ahlzén is working part-time as a general practitioner outside Karlstad in south-west Sweden. He is also the chairman of the ethical committee in the region of Värmland. He holds a position as senior lecturer in public health at Karlstad University, focusing mainly on healthcare ethics and on the history of ideas and science.

Martyn Evans joined Durham University in 2002 as Professor of Humanities in Medicine and Principal of John Snow College, and became Principal of Trevelyan College in 2008. He taught philosophy and ethics of medicine at the University of Wales for several years.

He was founding joint editor of the *Medical Humanities* edition of the *Journal of Medical Ethics* from 2000 to 2008. He has published variously on the aesthetics of music, ethics and philosophy of medicine, and the role of humanities in medical education. His current interests include music and medicine, the nature and role of humanities in medicine, and philosophical problems in medicine. In 2005 he was made an honorary Fellow of the Royal College of General Practitioners.

Pekka Louhiala is a lecturer in medical ethics at the University of Helsinki, Finland. He has degrees in both medicine and philosophy, and he also works as a part-time paediatrician in private practice. He has published on various topics in medical ethics, philosophy of medicine and epidemiology. His current academic interests include conceptual and philosophical issues in medicine, such as evidence-based medicine and placebo effects.

Raimo Puustinen is a full-time general practitioner and a senior consultant at Pihlajalinna Medical Centre, Tampere, Finland. He has published articles and books on general practice, medical ethics and philosophy of medicine. When not practising medicine or contemplating theoretical issues in medical practice, he tries to play jazz with tenor saxophone. He is married, and has four children and two grandchildren.

List of contributors

Jill Gordon
Honorary Associate Professor, Centre for Values Ethics and the Law in Medicine, University of Sydney

Iona Heath
General practitioner, Kentish Town, London

Jyrki Korkeila
Professor of Psychiatry, University of Turku, Finland
Consultant, Harjavalta Hospital, Satakunta Hospital District, Finland

Anne MacLeod
Dermatologist and writer from the North of Scotland

Jane Macnaughton
Director of the Centre for Arts and Humanities in Health and Medicine (CAHHM)
Clinical Senior Lecturer, Durham University

Carl-Edvard Rudebeck
Research Adviser, Kalmar County Council
Professor, Institute for Community Medicine, Tromsö University, Norway
General practitioner, Esplanaden Health Centre, Västervik

John Saunders
Honorary Professor, Centre for Philosophy, Humanities and Law in Healthcare, School of Health Science, University of Wales, Swansea
Honorary Senior Lecturer, College of Medicine, University of Wales, Cardiff
Consultant Physician, Nevill Hall Hospital, Abergavenny

Acknowledgements

The Editors of this second volume of *Medical Humanities Companion* again want to thank Radcliffe Publishing for its continued belief in this project. We are also very thankful for the support that we have received from the Signe and Ane Gyllenberg Foundation, who funded our meeting in Hämeenlinna in Finland, where the shape of this book took its final form. Finally, it has also been a pleasure for us to have Professor Jyrki Korkeila as guest contributor.

Introduction

When someone falls ill, the experiences of this person are changed. It might be a very minor and very transient change, or it may be decisive and lasting. What happens must be understood and most understanding takes place in language. Diagnosis is a word for what is happening to the ill person. It is to this naming of the illness experience and the bodily changes that often accompany it that this second volume of *Medical Humanities Companion* is dedicated.

In Volume One of this series, we explored the different meanings of symptoms. Fundamental to our efforts was the conviction that, as the editors expressed it, our task was to 'take seriously the patient's *subjectivity*'. Symptoms strike us as being exactly subjective, so there is, no doubt, subjectivity to attend to when these are expressed. But what about diagnosis? Isn't that something objective, or at least highly intersubjective? Diagnoses are associated to medical science, and science is allegedly based on facts established by rigorous methods. As a consequence, do we here move from the uncertain and vague terrain of subjectivity to the clear air of precise science?

One of our central aims in this second volume is to show that such assumptions are too simple. By casting light from different directions on the notion of diagnosis, we hope to make visible the complexities and ambiguities involved in giving and receiving diagnoses, as well as their socio-cultural background and consequences. Diagnoses, it will be seen, are powerful tools for good and bad. They shape and are shaped by our views on what is real, what is acceptable and how we relate to certain phenomena. Diagnoses are born and they die in a complex interaction between scientific discoveries, social negotiation and historical change.

A diagnosis is an answer to the human need that springs from being ill. To make this assertion into flesh and blood, into concrete human suffering, we start also this volume with the stories about five fictionalised persons – Rachel, Jake, Liz, Geoff and Jen – who are ill and who are about to receive their diagnoses. The fates of these persons are unique, and yet, we hope, in some way illuminating for the condition of being vulnerable and in need of qualified medical help. The individuals may hopefully serve as reminders that however important it is to analyse medicine on a general, abstract level, it is after all the needs of concrete human beings that are the very reason for there to be a science and a practice of medicine at all.

Finally, we want to repeat the last words from the introduction to the first volume: 'We do not know exactly where our patients' journeys will lead them, nor where our own enquiries will lead us. However, we hope to accompany them to their destinations, and we hope that our readers in turn will accompany us.'

Rolf Ahlzén
Martyn Evans
Pekka Louhiala
Raimo Puustinen
April 2010

CHAPTER 1

Narratives

ANNE MACLEOD

RACHEL

It didn't worry me when the doctor sat down on the bed and told me that from now on I would need to take care of myself. She said I would be fine, absolutely fine. As long as I tested my blood and had an injection – *two* injections – every single day.

Of course it worried me – can't you tell when I'm being brave? It's me I'm talking about – me – who's so frightened of injections I once refused to go to school because I knew the school nurse was coming in that day and someone had told me (it wasn't true) that every time she came she had a needle in her bag, big as your arm. Might have been Leroy who told me. Probably it was. When the doctor explained what was wrong with me – all the sugar stuff – all I could see in my head was that nurse's needle.

'You're a smart girl,' the doctor nodded. She was the youngest doctor in the ward. She always looked tired. Her hair was scruffed up in a clip at the back of her head. The loose bits bobbled as she moved around. She waved her hands a lot. 'It won't make you any different. You'll be able to do everything you want to do,' she said. 'Just like before. Being diabetic doesn't mean you have to change your dreams.'

'Diabetic? I'm a *diabetic*?' The word rang in my head like a hard, cold bell. 'Will I have to go a special school?

'Of course not,' the doctor smiled. 'You'll learn to manage. I'll come back and talk to you again, and Dax, our special diabetic nurse, will come and talk to you. And to your mother.'

'Mum knows?'

'Yes. She asked me to have this chat with you. She's outside now. With your brother.'

The doctor stood up and turned. She opened the door. I was still feeling wobbly when Mum came through. I could tell she'd been crying. I always know. The white bit of her eyes goes all red and her skin is always bumpy for hours.

'Hey Mum,' I said before her tears could fall. 'What took you so long? Where you been? Did you bring that new CD I asked for?'

That switched her into MUM mode. She glowered at me.

'Think I'm made of money, girl?'

Leroy sidled in behind her. It was the first time he'd come to see me. That boy is so scared of hospitals. And needles. And being sick. He looked at me with narrow eyes, like he was afraid if he opened them any more he might see something he didn't want to know. Like I might be an alien.

'Hey Leroy!'

'Hey sis–'

His high five was feeble. The drip thing in my arm seemed to put him off.

'I know. The doctor told me.' I glared at both them. 'About the injections and all. She says there's a special nurse coming to see me. Says I'll get to go to summer camp. Haven't I always wanted to go to summer camp?'

Leroy swallowed hard.

'Sis,' he said, 'I once read this book about a summer camp. It wasn't so good. They made these boys who hadn't done nothing in the first place dig holes five feet wide and five feet deep. That's the stuff you do at summer camp.'

'Not my camp.'

He didn't read that book. He asked me to read it for him so he could tell the teacher all about it. The book was called Holes. Thinking of it made me feel a little bit uncomfortable. I *would* be digging holes every day – not five feet wide, not in earth – holes in my own skin.

But they would keep me well, stop me being sick. I would be digging holes and filling them.

Leroy didn't stay long. Mum sent him to the cafe. Before she left, she gave me the biggest hug. I could feel an ocean of worry in her.

'Why did this have to happen to us?'

'I'll be fine, Mum. We'll be fine. This isn't the olden days.'

She pulled herself together. 'Course not,' she sniffed. 'What else did the doctor say?'

'Didn't she talk to you?'

'I couldn't take it all in. Not a thing.'

Mum sank back into silence. That was scary. I've never known Mum to sit so still. So quiet. I didn't know what to do with her. That was when the door opened again and Dax came in.

JAKE

The surgery wasn't in the same place any more. That was the first shock. Jake stood outside the building where it used to be. Fortunately there was still a sign explaining it had moved. Six months before. The sign was still there, still just about legible. He'd have to run though, to make his appointment time. The new place wasn't far away, but he only had ten minutes to get there. He was sweaty and breathless when he arrived.

The new place was all glass and wood. Doors swished aside as Jake approached. The receptionist behind the high pale counter looked over her glasses at him. 'Yes?'

'Jake Bryan. Appointment with Dr Siddha. Twelve fifteen.'

The receptionist's eyes swung to the clock. Twelve eighteen. Jake was late.

'Take a seat. Dr Siddha is running over time.'

She was. At five to one, Jake, finding himself alone in the waiting room, approached the desk once more.

'Excuse me–'

The receptionist drew her eyes away, reluctantly, it seemed to Jake, from the fascinations of the screen before her.

'I had an appointment with Dr Siddha.'

'Twelve fifteen.'

'Only she hasn't called me yet. Is she still here?'

'Her surgery is running late.'

'How late?' Jake blushed. 'Only I'm due at work at two.'

'Take a seat.' The receptionist glanced back at the screen. 'You're next. It won't be long.'

Twenty minutes later, an apprehensive Jake eased himself back on to the chair facing the doctor. His heart was thumping. He found it hard to concentrate. He wasn't used to displaying his body. Hated it. Worse, he had not expected the intrusion of what the doctor had called the rectal examination.

'Sorry to do this,' she'd apologised. 'But with that history of blood in the bowel movements, we'd better get it over. Just relax. Deep breaths now – there you go–'

He had never imagined anything like this. His cheeks were burning. Answering the questions had been bad enough, all that *blood in the bowel movements*, but this–

'Fine. Get dressed. We'll have a talk about things.'

As he pulled his clothes on he heard her peeling off the rubber gloves, washing her hands, pulling a paper towel from the dispenser by the sink. Not comfortable noises. Her feet clumped over to the desk and he was aware of her sliding the mouse across the desktop.

'Come and sit down when you're ready.' Dr Siddha seemed unworried, as if this were an ordinary everyday thing. 'Good. Nothing to worry about. Nothing at all. The proctoscopy – the examination of the back passage shows a minor problem with haemorrhoids. Most lay people would call them piles. You've heard of those, yes?' Her eyes rested on him, briefly. 'But there's nothing else abnormal to be seen there. We can do one of two things – either watch the situation, see how you get on over the next few weeks and months, or perhaps try something simple like peppermint oil, assuming your symptoms have been caused by a minor dysfunction of the bowel we call Irritable Bowel Syndrome. Or–'

'Or?' Jake nodded, miserable.

'Or,' Dr Siddha continued, 'we could send you up to the hospital for further tests.'

'Tests?' Jake's throat was sandpaper.

'Colonoscopy, perhaps. Nothing too invasive.'

'Colonoscopy?' Jake was aware he had turned into an echo. 'What's that?'

Dr Siddha was writing in his notes.

'They pass a tube,' she said, 'into the bowel and examine it directly, a little like we did today.'

Jake didn't like the sound of that. 'Could we try the oil first?'

'Certainly. Your problems certainly tick all the boxes for IBS.'

'IBS.' Jake thought that sounded like a computer.

'Irritable Bowel Syndrome.' Dr Siddha clicked her mouse and the printer on her desk began to hum. 'Here,' she handed him the newly typed prescription, and a larger sheet of paper. 'Here's some information for you. Come back if these don't help, or if things get worse. Don't exceed the stated dose. Have you any questions?'

Jake shook his head.

'What about the psoriasis? Can I help you with that?'

Jake had had enough for one day. 'No problems there.' He had almost reached the door. 'Thank you, Doctor Siddha.'

'No problem,' she sighed, dismissing him. 'Take care, now.'

LIZ

Some days the dropping of the mail on the doormat feels promising, positive. Other days the clustered envelopes, both brown and white, look dull at best – or worse, intrusive. That morning, Liz was later than she'd hoped to be. Less organised. She should not have turned over and gone back to sleep after the alarm. Yes, her cases were packed. Yes, Sophie was ready too, all brushed and neat in her best holiday clothes. Yes, she'd checked the house. Doors and windows locked, plugs pulled out, switches off. Sophie had taken the cat food out of the utility room and left it in the shed for Izzie, who was going to feed the animals over the holiday. The taxi was due in less than five minutes.

Liz realised she had not packed her tablets, or her toothbrush, for that matter. She rushed upstairs. When she came down again, the mail lay on the carpet. Sophie picked it up.

'Shall I leave this in the kitchen, Mum?'

'No, give it here. We've time.'

Liz regretted asking for the mail. Regretted opening that letter. An invitation, it said, to return for a further smear test. Her last sample, it trilled, unemotionally, had been either insufficient, or shown minor abnormalities. She had just finished reading when the taxi came.

She dumped the sheaf of letters on the hallstand. If she'd been thinking straight, she would have stuffed that one in her over-full bag. She was in the taxi, almost at the airport before the message hit home. Her smear had shown minor abnormalities. What did that mean? What could it mean? Cancer? Infection?

Carlos slept around at the end of their relationship. He always denied it, but Liz knew. She had asked the doctor then to screen her for infection. All the tests were negative. Surely there could not be repercussions now?

And if not infection, what then?

'Mum? When we get there, let's go straight to the beach. Before unpacking.'

'It might be raining, Soph.'

'You say that every year. It never rains. If it does we could go to the Quernstone instead.'

'You do that every year. You love that shop. Funny that you always forget your purse.'

Traditional holiday banter. Liz was on auto-pilot, one word pounding her brain. Cancer. *Cancer*. **Cancer**.

'Mum! What is it with you today?'

'Sorry?'

'Our flight's delayed. Look at the screen. No point in going to the gate for an least an hour.'

Liz sighed. That was all she needed. They went for a drink, wasted time in the airport shops. Sophie tried on scarves, gauzy caftans. She, at least, was having fun.

'What d'you think Mum?'

Liz found she could not join in, could not concentrate. She felt sick. Her hands were shaking. She must do something now or the worry would over-whelm the holiday. Stress set her fits off too. She came to a sudden decision.

'Look Soph, mind the bags, will you? I've a call to make.'

She could not go away with this hanging over her head, this sword of Damocles. So she found a quiet corner, took out her phone and dialled. The electronic system, baffling as ever, wafted her through to – at last – a human voice.

'How may I help you?'

Liz explained.

'I know Dr Wocjik won't be free, but I wondered when I might call her back?'

'Actually, she's just come off a call. I'll put you through.'

'Liz–' Dr Wocjik's voice was light and clear, 'an abnormal smear, you say – let me get this up on the screen.

'Ah – and you've been worrying: I can hear it in your voice. Where are you? At the airport? Going where? The Orkneys? Marvellous. I hear it's wonderful up there.

'Sorry to take so long. The machines are slow today.

'Right. Here we are. Look Liz, as far as I can see, this is just an insufficient smear. We ought to repeat it. You weren't so well that day. Are things better on that front? Good. Now, what I want to say, Liz, is – enjoy your holiday. Make an appointment with me when you come back and I'll repeat the test.

'Don't waste time worrying, The screening we do picks up a range of things – chlamydia, for example. You've heard of that? – Most people know about it these days – or early changes that might represent untidiness in the cervical lining cells. It is certainly worth repeating the test again, but let me emphasise again – from what I have here, there's no clear cause for worry. No definite diagnosis. Insufficient evidence, that's all.

'Is that helpful? Is there anything else you want to ask me? Anything at all? No? Right. Will I give you back to Jane now to make that appointment? Or would you rather phone when you get home? Take the day off work. It will be less stressful that way. Easier than last time.'

Liz snapped her phone shut. Closed her eyes, shaking with relief.

'Mum! Mum! Where have you been? Haven't you been listening to the announcements? What have you been doing? Our flight is boarding *now*. They're calling our names. Come on! Let's go – Mum!'

JEN AND GEOFF

Sometimes travelling on a bus makes Jen feel good: young again. Makes her think of the days when Geoff was young and strong. Didn't he look handsome in his driver's uniform? And she'd looked fine as well, smart as a new pin, that's what everybody always said. No other clippie came close. Jen strode the decks of her double-decker dealing out tickets, gathering fares, and all the local gossip. All the gen. Today, though, the bus ride hasn't been so good. Not like the old days.

It's not the same flashing your bus-pass on the way in.

It was good of Dr Gaitens to organise a lady from Crossroads to sit with Geoff while she went to the clinic. The hospital's a long way off: two bus journeys. They don't have a car, not any more, and Jen never did learn to drive. Never felt the lack of it, not till Geoff's stroke. Till then they did everything together.

Not any more. She's managed though. Done everything. Maybe that's why she's been so short of energy, tired all the time.

And she's not sleeping well. How would you? Didn't she remember what her brother Albert went through when he started coughing blood? All those months in hospital away from everyone; sleeping outside in the snow on a verandah. In the end they even collapsed one of his lungs! Till Bert died he'd looked too thin and a bit crooked.

The hospital is different too. Much larger. Not all the changes are bad though. For one thing, waiting in outpatients isn't what it used to be. She remembers rows and rows of folk marooned there for whole afternoons, sitting in surgical gowns and rough striped dressing gowns woven, it seemed, from pipe cleaners. Now the waiting room is smarter, and the dressing gowns have been banished to the cavernous changing rooms of Outpatient X-ray. The robe they give her swamps her. Everything does that these days; since Geoff's stroke – what with all the extra work – she's turning into Twiggy.

It's raining. Jen traces the raindrops on the bus window. Thinking of the clinic. Of Dr Murray looking at her, saying something quiet, about a shadow on the X-ray. Jen burst into tears. She's always been afraid of those words. Shadow. On. The X. Ray.

Her mother died of TB. Bert didn't, though. Despite the years in hospital, Bert didn't die of TB in the end. Killed in a car accident.

'It's TB, is it Doctor?'

The doctor shook his head. 'No, not TB. That would be most unlikely.'

Dr Murray is nice, tall and thin. He'd look good in a smart coat. He'd look good in tails. His white coat is too small for him, the arms too short. He's speaking to her. Still speaking. 'Not TB. A different sort of shadow. We need to do more tests, then work out a treatment plan. Cancer is a possibility. Did you ever smoke, Mrs Doughty?'

Her head is spinning. All those years she'd forced herself to smoke! She hadn't even liked it. She doesn't like it now, but never managed to stop.

A treatment plan.

Jen feels cold. And sick. The bus ride is not helping, jolting her along through the dark streets and bright lights. Everything seems unreal. It's taking her – where? Not home, surely. She'd better, she thinks, phone Mark and Mary – her son, Geoff's daughter. But not today. Not today. It'll be bad enough not telling Geoff.

No point in telling him. He wouldn't take it in.

And what if it turns out to be TB after all? What could she tell him then?

GEOFF

Dr Gaitens was so good on the phone, reassuring.

'We'll do what we can,' he assured her. 'Access all the help they need when they need it.'

Mary was not so sure now that things would be so simple. She'd spent three days with her father, three days while his wife, her stepmother Jen, lingered in the Chest and Infectious Diseases Unit of Killen Hospital. Jen, Mary could see, was losing weight. Fast.

Geoff never had been easy, but the stroke had left him in the worst of all worlds, immobile and angry. Jen seems to cope, but Mary could not imagine how. Her stepmother's strength of character, her selfless devotion to the wheelchair-bound, cantankerous dictator Geoff had somehow morphed into, was hard to compute.

For the last three days, since Jen left, he had not said a word. Not a word. He had eaten nothing. None of the meals Mary cooked for him. Jen had left a list of what he would and would not take. He did not eat. Would not even drink. He sat staring into space, a shrunken version of himself. Mary panicked, phoned the surgery again.

It was five o'clock when Dr Gaitens arrived, after his surgery.

'How's your mother?'

'Jen, you mean? Geoff's wife?'

'She's not your mother?' Dr Gaitens followed her along the narrow hall. Mary was ashamed of the paintwork, so badly scratched by the wheelchair. She meant to patch it up.

'My mother died when I was seventeen.' Her voice, despite her best intentions, shrivelled, grew cold. 'He moved her in before the month was out. Jen's not my mother.'

Dr Gaitens did not even blink, turned into the bedroom.

'Well, Geoff? And how are you today?'

His questions drew no more response than Mary's ranting. Geoff ignored them all. After a good twenty minutes, Dr Gaitens found his way back to the kitchen where Mary was drinking tea, staring out across the pin-neat garden.

'He always loved his garden,' she nodded.

'Who keeps it now?'

'She does. Before the stroke he never let her touch a thing in it. Told her she hadn't a green bone in her body.' She looked directly at the doctor. 'How is he?'

'Profoundly depressed. Of course, he has been for some time, but he's much worse. Somewhat dehydrated too. Missing your stepmother. Any further news from the hospital?'

Mary shrugged. 'She hasn't taken it in. They think it's cancer. They seem almost sure. What they can do about it depends on the tests they're doing now. What about Dad? He can't stay here.'

'No.' Dr Gaitens agrees. 'It's been touch and go for months. When are you expecting Jen home?'

Mary looks blank.

'They didn't say. But I've to be back south by Friday at the latest. I can't stay any longer. He needs proper care.'

'I'll try Geriatrics. The assessment unit,' Dr Gaitens frowned. 'They're busy, though. Don't get your hopes too high. If you'll excuse me–'

Mary strained to hear him in the hall, but the words ran into each other, indistinct. He knocked on the kitchen door before coming back in.

'Good news. They'll have a bed tomorrow. I'll organise an ambulance. We'll phone from the surgery to give you an approximate time for that. I'll just pop back and tell your father.'

Dr Gaitens spent the next five minutes explaining to Geoff what was happening, where he'd be. What the hospital was like. The things he'd need to pack. It irritated Mary, him wasting so much time. Geoff, staring at the wall, didn't seem to hear.

CHAPTER 2

Diagnosis: an introduction

ROLF AHLZÉN

FROM SYMPTOM TO DIAGNOSIS

Symptoms are bodily sensations or mental states that call for medical help. The complexity of symptoms – how they are experienced, interpreted and handled by ill persons, relatives and doctors – has been explored in Volume One, *Symptom*, of the *Medical Humanities Companion*. The contributors to this first volume all, in different ways, illuminated the unwished, intruding, obstructive character of most symptoms. Symptoms call for explanation. They call for naming. They call for understanding and a path to recovery, back to one's 'usual' self, like coming back 'home'. Almost all who fall ill want a diagnosis. This gives at least a hope for recovery. The symptoms may with a diagnosis acquire meaning, though often enough brittle and provisional. The path to diagnosis and recovery generally involves the physician, in case of more severe illness. 'The doctor is the person who takes the history', in Stephen Toulmin's words. The doctor is also most often the person who – with the crucial help of the story of the illness – makes the diagnosis, although others such as the ill person herself, relatives, and friends may make their own conjectures. We turn our attention to this process in this second volume. In what follows, some aspects of these richly complex phenomena will be introduced. They are all connected, more or less explicitly, to the narratives that precede this introduction. After symptoms, diagnosis is the focus of our efforts to understand what the practice of medicine is about.

BEING ILL AND HAVING A DISEASE

A diagnosis is the name of a disease. When I have been given a diagnosis, I have a disease. The disease is in some strange way in my body, has 'come into it'. It may go away by itself or it may be made to go away by the measures taken by, usually, a doctor – and more or less as a consequence of my own efforts. Of course, it may not go away at all: it may become a permanent resident, like an intruder that sees my body as his new home – and, in doing so, makes my body alien and unreliable.

Of course, nowadays we know that diseases are not strange powers taking control over our bodies. From an early age we have been taught that diseases arise inside the body, that they are deviances of bodily function, that they can be described and measured and given names through scientific methods. We should know this modern lesson, but do we? Are we through and through 'modern' in our ways of feeling and thinking about our own diseases? If someone's body feels like jelly, if he suffers from a fatigue that permeates all his thoughts and movements, if he is just not able to do almost any of the things he would wish to do – may we then expect him to look at this as a localised biomedical deviance arising in some tissue of his body? It doesn't seem likely, except perhaps during short glimpses of reflection. Would he not rather experience his disease as an alteration of his bodily being *as a whole*? At times, he might think it came from 'somewhere', 'arose' somewhere in the body – but the illness itself has taken a hold over his entire being. In a way, falling ill gives rise to two ways of experiencing, relying simultaneously on internalised and scientifically based popular notions (that diseases arise in parts of the body that do not function as they should), and on age-old ways of apprehending afflictions. The latter may seem 'magical', equating the disease with some alien power that has taken hold of me as a whole and is plaguing me as if to punish me.

Doctors diagnose and fight diseases. They need diagnoses to find out why, to be able to speak of and compare, to find remedies and to make conjectures about the future. If there is no diagnosis, there is nothing apart from symptoms to fight against. The evil remains nameless. The diagnosis makes the state of the person into *something*. It becomes tangible, graspable, fightable. Without a diagnosis, the symptoms will remain mysterious and meaningless for the afflicted person. The diagnosis is a blessing and, in case it is a serious disease, also a curse.

As explored in Volume One of this series, it is the unwanted sensations and perceptions that we call symptoms that bring the ill person to the physician.[1]

These perceptions may be distressing in themselves (ache, itching, dizziness, panic) and hence create a wish for relief; or they may not be particularly unpleasant (a lump in the breast, a strange rash) but rather worrying, pointing to something that might become very unpleasant. All sorts of questions will arise: 'What is this, will it go away, who will make it go away, how long is it going to take, what will they do . . . IS IT DANGEROUS?' Diagnosis is usually the first and crucial step towards a way out of this alien chaos of unanswered questions.

A diagnosis is hence not only a label for a disease, whether experienced as a foreign invader or thought of as a physico-chemical deviance. It is also a name for a condition, for a predicament, for an existential situation. Being ill, I am no longer myself, something 'is the matter'. I don't feel the way that I want to feel, my plans are obstructed. I do not feel 'at home' any more. This is a strictly personal experience, possibly one of the most personal of all. Giving it the same general label as is given to similar conditions in other people, certainly says *something* about it, but does it say very much? The name of the disease, the diagnosis, makes an abstraction of all uniquely personal aspects and focuses on the common traits that unite this individual's condition with a number of other individuals' conditions. The ill person feels that he is like them – but knows that he is not quite like them. My rheumatoid arthritis is mine, and yours is yours. Still, both the ill person and the doctor (and a number of other professionals) need the diagnosis.

DO DISEASES EXIST?

As Jyrki Korkeila reminds us in his essay on psychiatric diagnoses, giving labels is a basic human activity. By naming things we orient ourselves in the world and try to understand and master them. Labels refer to patterns. They create categories under which unique phenomena may be grouped. But names not only depict existing reality, they create new realities. We see through the prism of concepts. Hence, when doctors group some collection of symptoms together and give them a name, do they then also 'invent' a new disease?

Let's take an example. Did hyperactivity disorders among children, for example the DAMP or ADHD syndromes, *exist* in any reasonable meaning of this word forty years ago? In one way, it seems as if the disease really was there before. As I recall some of my schoolmates in the late fifties, it seems obvious. Surely one or two of them had DAMP/ADHD. But did they really, as these categories were not used at that time? Before there is a name to it, in what sense is it there? The question is a philosophical one, but the way we answer it will have important consequences for how we consider and manage similar problems. To put it another way: is the increased diagnosis of these children an expression of medicine's sharp observing eye, with resulting options of acknowledgment and relief to distressed families? Or is it an expression of the growing medicalisation of western societies, where more and more deviations from the normal acquire diagnostic labels, become 'pathologised' and are seen as objects for medical interventions? May it even be both?

Critical questions about diagnostic habits are posed by social constructivists, who, as self-appointed advocates of the long nominalist tradition in western philosophy,[2] emphasise the fact that diseases and diagnoses come and go. Sociologists tell us we should search for the social forces governing such processes, which cannot be expected to be entirely benevolent. Some of them conclude that diseases are invented, 'constructed', under the pressure of cultural and historical conditions, for reasons of power, of control, of socio-economic adaptation. In this way, social scientists may challenge physicians and show them who have the tools for *really* understanding these phenomena. Physicians, and their medical science, are naïve, constructivists would have it, when they make us believe that diseases exist the way you and I, or stones or aircrafts, exist.

We need not dwell long on this. The discussion is old and will not be solved here. One reason for this is that both sides have a point. Of course diagnoses are relative to time and culture: how could they be otherwise? One need not be an anthropologist to acknowledge the variety of conceptions of illness among cultures in the world; nor does one need to be an historian to understand that diagnoses depend on historical factors. But there is more to be said. Diagnoses do come and go, we do change our view of what is healthy and what is ill, of how persons get ill, and what can cure them. This can hardly mean that *diseases*, as biological and existential phenomena, are invented or constructed, in the ordinary sense of these words. It seems more reasonable to say that our ways of thinking about them, of interpreting them, are in some sense 'constructed', even though such a choice of words may imply too much deliberation and purpose.

The biological as well as mental realities that constitute what we call illness and disease are real enough; they *are* really there in the most urgent way possible. It is our understanding of them that is continually changed, just as our understanding of what goes on inside and outside of us changes continuously. It is seriously misleading to say that we go about 'constructing' the world around us.[3] The world is there and we incessantly keep on interpreting it. In the same way, diseases are there before our interpretation of them. For young Rachel in our narrative, her diabetes is overwhelmingly real, and it would surely strike her and her relatives as exceedingly odd to say that the disease is 'constructed'.

WHY DIAGNOSIS?

It has been noted above that diagnoses are important for patients as well as healthcare professionals. For the ill person, a diagnosis carries the potential for answering three questions, crucial for anyone who gets symptoms that are more than transient and that worry and obstruct:

> What is this, what is happening in my body?

> Why did I get it, where does it come from?

> What can be done about it, will it heal by itself or must something be done in order to get rid of it?

As we will see, few of our present diagnoses can answer all these questions. Either we do not know the aetiology of the disease, what caused it, or we do not really understand what is happening in the body (the pathophysiology), or both. In addition, we are often unable to cure it and can only modify its course, valuable though that may be. The success of modern medicine will of course depend on its degree of control over the course of diseases. To cure, to alleviate, or to console – these are the goals and they are all served by diagnoses.

These questions above cannot be answered fully from the biomedical perspective. The second question, the crucial 'why', is a biomedical why *and* an existential why. It is dangerous to misunderstand these two aspects of the ill person, and mix them up with each other. Practitioners of medicine may believe that the biomedical answer ('You got this disease because you smoked and ate fatty food and this led to a process in your coronary arteries that made them too narrow . . .') is the full answer. Conversely, advocates of, for example, new-age inspired theories of diseases may believe that the existential answer ('You got this disease because you have lost contact with your deeper spirituality and lost yourself') is all that is needed.

One may object that doctors do indeed not always think and act like that, and also that there really are people for whom the existential 'why' is not interesting. They are content to look at disease, including their own, as a purely biomedical phenomenon and remain genuinely uninterested in whatever 'meaning' the disease may have from whatever perspective. From this point of view it could be said that the 'meaning' of the disease is that it is there – devoid of any meaning, just arbitrary and pointing to nothing beyond itself. Many people may think this way and to say that they have a reduced or impoverished understanding of their illness – as is occasionally done – would be foolish. Perhaps they should even be congratulated for being courageous enough to see diseases for what they really are: meaningless biological incidents, motors of evolution, just as alien to human morality and meaning as the winds blowing over the oceans or the stars wandering in the night sky?

An ill person becomes more estranged from himself, if the illness intrudes and persists. The ill person becomes excluded from many of the contexts that constituted her everyday life. Diagnosis can create a partially changed identity and perhaps a new belonging. When there is a name for the disease, there are also others who 'have it'. There is a community of sufferers. There are things to read about it and stories to listen to. The welfare system, if there is one, will welcome you as a legitimate receiver of support. People around you will usually show compassion and consideration. In this way, diagnoses may help to make life more 'homelike' again, even if the home is not quite the same any more.

The capacity to adjust to and come to terms with illness is, however, not an uncomplicated blessing. Illness creates identity and a sort of meaning for some. May it be that persons whose lives are very far from 'homelike', who feel deserted and hopeless and unrecognised, may unconsciously wish to be diagnosed with 'something' that makes their lives meaningful again, or at least bearable? Physician Olle Hellström has written about this in an interesting way, in articles on patients with fibromyalgia.[4] Hellström argues that if these persons are helped to find a more constructive way to find meaning in their lives, the symptoms will go away. However, accepting this possibility does not mean that doctors should jump to premature conclusions about the reasons why people become ill.

Let us stop for a while to look at our narratives. Rachel gets her diagnosis after some time. It is a precise diagnosis of a very well known condition. She is told that she has diabetes, a disease that in spite of progress in treatment still carries serious consequences and therefore sounds threatening to many people. Is she relieved? Is she confused? Is she shocked? Is she hopeful? She may be all these things at the same time. Diabetes is a chronic disease, but one for which she will get good help to master. Had Rachel lived in the early 20th century, it would have killed her within a rather short time. The diagnosis would have been a verdict with no escape. In the 21st century, Rachel will be a 'diabetic', but she and everyone around her know that this means relatively little to her chances to lead a fulfilled life, although the long term consequences are problematic. Gradually, Rachel will know and understand that there is likely to be a toll taken by the disease, however well she manages to control it.

Doctors, too, need diagnoses. They would be powerless if all cases were unique and if no knowledge could be gained on a general level from particular cases. Only by inferring from generalised knowledge about a disease category to a specific case in that category can physicians decide on treatment. This is a complicated step. Diagnoses are important tools for physicians, but diagnoses also exert power over doctors. Diagnostic thinking is like a filter in front of the physician's eyes, including and excluding, guiding what she sees or does not see, what she searches for or does not search for, asks or does not ask. We know from several studies that doctors tend to jump to diagnostic conclusions too early in the diagnostic process.[5] Like a bell ringing at the back of the physician's head, saying 'pneumonia' over and over again, it numbs other voices that might whisper 'pulmonary embolism' or 'pleuritis' or 'asthma'. It furthermore might wipe away those voices that try to tell the doctor that there are other things here to attend to, a person in despair, a human being reaching out for mutual human understanding, for something to hope for in a life with too little hope.

Byron Good has shown, in his seminal study from Harvard medical school, how medical students become more and more focused on diagnosing disease. One student is quoted as expressing his ambition this way:

> You are not there just to talk with people and learn about their lives and nurture them. You're not there for that. You're a professional and you're trained in interpreting phenomenological descriptions of behavior into physiologic and pathophysiologic processes.[6]

Of course, one may remark, isn't that indeed what he *is* there for? Who else, but the physician could infer from personal experience (symptom) to biomedical deviance? But, on the other hand, if the student does not, when he starts practising as doctor, realise that if he *only* translates from the biographical to the scientific and if he thus looks upon his patient's words exclusively as a tool to reach the real thing, the disease – then he is bound to get into trouble and will not be able either to diagnose nor treat patients in an intelligent and respectful manner. If the focus of physicians exclusively is on what Martyn Evans calls 'the medicalised body'[7] and if their gaze is only working in an 'objectifying' way, we are again facing the question of how the person shall be seen, recognised, and confirmed by this scientifically trained eye?

Diagnosis is powerful. It filters and sorts, it directs conclusions, it governs emotions and delivers self-reinforcing chains of actions. Awareness of this fact may lead to caution and temperance. It is a bit like dealing with explosive material. It may be extremely useful for many beneficial purposes but must be handled with restraint and with well developed precautions.

REACHING DIAGNOSIS

Diagnosis is sometimes the result of investigations that precede it.[8] This phase may be swift and precise or drawn out and undirected. Many of the symptoms prompting patients to seek help are so vague that they point in many possible directions. Furthermore, the same symptom or sign – for example, Jake's stains of blood in the stool – may point to a serious disorder, like cancer of the rectum, but in most cases be innocent enough – as it seems in Jake's case. The diagnostic ambition will then be to exclude the dangerous alternatives with sufficient certainty, and then treat the minor condition. As for Jake, the whole diagnostic procedure may be stressful, associated with shyness, shame and worry. Diagnosis will then be a relief, both because it marks the end of the investigations and also because it, if it points to the easily curable, resolves worry and fear.

The period of diagnostic procedures – whether short or extended – is a delicate phase of dialogue between doctor and patient. How may a physician wisely handle the responsibility to keep her patient informed of what is going on in an investigation where there is some degree of suspicion that there may be a serious disease present? Jen's doctor has seen 'a shadow' on her chest X-ray. Jen fears that it might be tuberculosis – obviously from her early life experiences of this – but the doctor flatly declares that 'cancer is a possibility'. Of course, Jen's head then goes into a spin. A diagnostic suspicion is presented in a rather brutal way, without any qualification, any interest in Jen's reaction and no chance of hope for another outcome. The built in reservation – '. . . is a possibility' – can hardly be expected to relieve Jen very much. Should it later turn out that she does not, after all, have either cancer or TB, she has been worried in an unnecessary way. Being truthful about diagnostic procedures does not mean being insensitive and discouraging.

Modern medicine has created new kinds of diagnostic situations. Traditionally, people sought medical help when they were feeling unwell and thought that this was for reasons that a doctor – or other healer – could do something about. This is, of course, still most often the case. But medical technologies have now opened up the body for investigation. Asymptomatic persons come to doctors to be 'checked', and some deviance from the normal is then detected. Typically, this may be an elevated blood pressure, a cervical smear with atypical cells, suspect changes on a breast X-ray, high blood cholesterol and/or glucose levels. Diagnosis here acquires a partly different function. Today, almost everyone has been taught to be cautious, to go for medical 'control', so that no undetected process is going on in his or her body that might *in the long run* be harmful. For this reason patients are not always diagnosed or treated for what they feel and experience here and now, but for what they might, often with some degree of probability, come to experience in the future. Liz's chaotic feelings illustrate this. From a medical point of view, her fear is disproportionate. But Liz is not a doctor and it is her body, her future, which is at stake. She knows well enough that the smear is a test for early stages of cancer. How could she know that these early stages are very far from being developed cancers and that we do not even know if all early deviances would eventually develop into malignancies? In such a situation, it would be foolish to expect full rationality or knowledge from those who are diagnosed with a 'risk'.

Some years ago, Swedish anthropologist Lisbeth Sachs looked at a group of men receiving the diagnosis 'hyper-cholesterolemia' – that is, elevated blood concentrations of cholesterol. The men reacted very differently. Some were 'rational' in the sense that they really didn't worry very much, they were capable of seeing it as a low-grade, long-term risk that they could check with new habits, and perhaps medicine. But a number of them reacted with strong worry, grave uncertainty and fantasies about white projectiles rushing around in their blood stream ready to get stuck somewhere in the heart or brain. So, even if we lack large scale studies of patients' experiences of being diagnosed with 'risk factors', we have enough evidence to indicate that the search for hidden risk factors may have negative consequences. What is won in the prevention or postponement of disease may be lost in personal well-being, sense of security and trust.

THE FOUNDATIONS OF DIAGNOSIS

Modern diagnostic systems are oriented towards disease, not illness. Illness is subjective and the ill person is supremely knowledgeable about what it means to him or her. By contrast, it is the state of the medically described body that is usually the basis for a diagnosis. In medicine, there has been and still is a strong wish for diagnosis to be based on 'hard' findings, such as laboratory measurements or X-rays. This leaves us, however, with a challenge: if 'having a disease' is seen as the back-ground for 'being ill', and if illness is given limited relevance for diagnosis, is there a risk that personal experience is brushed aside by the physician? The ill person goes to see the doctor not because of some lesion in a part of his body, he goes there because he is worried, because he doesn't function and suffers from this. The doctor then looks for a lesion, a damage, a dysfunction, that *will explain* his ill-being. This will be the diagnosis. But what does it mean if no diagnosis is reached? If nothing is found? If all parameters, the hearts sounds, the abdominal ultrasound, the chest X-ray . . . if all these show nothing deviant, nothing out of order? Then there is no disease, is there? But *the patient does not feel well.* There might be a disease that can't be seen. So why not search more, even closer, make ever more complex investigations of his body? A diagnosis, after all, promises to rescue the patient from the territory of hopeless uncertainty to the solid ground of biomedical diagnosis and treatment. So, the search must go on . . ..

Let us speculate a little. With a system of diagnosis based on the illness experience this challenge would not arise. If someone experiences a stubborn pain in the arm, she would get a diagnosis that describes the kind of pain, say, 'VAS 7-pain in distal radial part of right forearm'.[9] This would turn the initial focus from disease to illness, but it would perhaps bring us into another dilemma, perhaps worse. Describing symptoms is just one step to cure. If we cannot through close investigation find a causal factor behind the pain, then what can we do about it? On the other hand, if we find a nerve entrapped the disease-based diagnosis will be 'Nerve entrapment of the radial nerve', the patient will be operated on and relieved of her pain.

But again: why would we necessarily need the biomedical localisation and/or pathophysiological characterisation already in the diagnosis? An experience-based diagnosis might be linked to biomedical physiology through our knowledge of common causal explanations for exactly this experience, in a second step. The pain in the arm, as defined by the person experiencing it, would then be followed by a number of hypotheses as to the cause of it. This is, of course, often how we actually work in hospitals and surgeries, when we don't know the biomedical background of illness experiences. Diagnosis based exclusively on symptom description is very common. But just as obvious is that the diagnosis 'Pain in forearm' is often seen by doctors as carrying less weight, indeed as having a lesser degree of reality, than 'Entrapment of radial nerve'.

Symptoms are often vague and surely not always a solid base for diagnoses. They are also by their very nature uniquely personal. A diagnosis based only on symptom presentation would, to be precise, mean one diagnosis for each ill person and the whole point of diagnosing would be lost. Fatigue, for example, is one of the most common symptoms leading people to seek medical help. Fatigue is almost always unlocalised, diffuse, hard to capture into words. 'Fatigue' as diagnosis says very little. Trying to overcome that dilemma would mean the opposite problem: a diagnosis based on the uniquely personal experience of fatigue is of no therapeutic value, because no general knowledge whatsoever would be applicable. The confirmation of the individual experience would perhaps be beneficial to the patient in one sense, but it would hardly help to cure the disease.

We meet the same difficulty when trying to find a general name for uniquely personal, strange and to most of us peculiar experiences, such as occur in some psychiatric illnesses. Depression, to take a very common example, is still a diagnosis made exclusively according to the ill person's unique personal experience of being in a very low mood, sleeping badly, losing appetite, experiencing guilt and inertia and lacking hope and joy. It is not diagnosed as 'Hypothalamic hyposerotonism', according to what seems to be a biochemical disturbance accompanying certain cases of depression. This may be because we simply lack a good way of measuring serotonin levels in specific parts of the brain, but it may also be that the whole idea of psychiatric illness is oriented towards experience. Most of us are probably inclined to say that in psychiatry, in contrast to somatic illness, the experience *is* the disease, whereas say, with a cardiac infarction it is certainly the thrombosis in the coronary artery that is seen as the real thing, and the chest pain a secondary phenomenon to this. (Some psychiatrists deplore this and would rather have psychiatric illness as a disease of the central nervous system, just like epilepsy or multiple sclerosis or Parkinson's disease). And there are exceptions. Trigeminal neuralgia and classical migraine, for example, produce such typical experiential features in the patient's symptom account that we consider them as somatic diseases, requiring neurologists, not psychiatrists.

THE GROWTH OF TAXONOMIES UP TO ICD-10

The wish for diagnosis is nothing new. We know from the history of medicine how over and over again attempts have been made to assemble and group conditions that make human beings suffer and prevent their functioning. The Hippocratic doctors were, seen in perspective, rather modest. With the advent of modern times, especially the 18th century, the systems – taxonomies, nomenclatures – grew exponentially. The nosographies of the 18th century bear witness to this. *Nosologhia methodica*, the most used of the classifications during the 18th century, mentions 2400 different diagnoses. By combining symptoms in intricate ways, the possibilities became almost endless.[10] Were there no medical signs, then? Indeed there were, but these were of a character-istically general kind, pointing to general states of the body, not localised (as there was no theory of how a localised pathological process could produce general symptoms and signs).

The rise of modern medicine has been closely associated with the devel-opment of more precise and systematic nomenclatures, usually based on pathophysiology. The ICD-10 now dominates throughout the world. It is gradually expanding, as new scientific knowledge is built into the system and as new conditions 'appear' as disease states. Meanwhile, other diagnoses disap-pear. The system now resembles a huge tree, spreading out into ever narrower branches. Some small branches disappear, while new ones appear. Out there, in the periphery, highly specialised clinicians make use of diagnoses that most often are unknown to the vast majority of other physicians. In renal medicine, for example, chronic inflammatory disease of the glomeruli of the kidney is now represented by eight different diagnoses, based on differences in pathol-ogy. No physician except the nephrologists needs to know very much about this, and GPs will usually consider only the larger diagnostic branch 'chronic glomerulonephritis'.

DIAGNOSTIC IMPERIALISM

The spread of diagnostic ambitions to new areas may be seen as an expression of an ongoing medicalisation of society. This phenomenon has been a constant theme in sociological literature during the last decades. Ivan Illich's critique of the tendency of modern medicine to infiltrate people's lives, from birth to death, though perhaps less discussed today than thirty years ago, remains both provoking and worrying.[11] In the sixties and seventies, psychiatric dia-gnosis was at the centre of this debate. Psychiatry was alleged to pathologise dissenters, making them into psychiatric cases so that the oppressive workings of capitalist society were hidden under medical diagnosis. Though it has not altogether disappeared, this critique has sunk into the background in favour of, for example, debates about physicians' and drug companies' alleged or real ambitions to spread diagnostic thinking and pharmacological treatment to new areas.

During the last decade it is the intensified search for risk factors that are possible to diagnose and treat that is being questioned. Some voices warn that medicine is gradually being transformed into a frantic search for minor risks, and that the drug industry, with the willing aid of doctors, uses our fear of disease and death to make whole populations dependent on their services. As these risks are gradually defined in ways that include larger and larger groups and as new drugs are developed that reduce the risk factor, the situation may indeed feed 'medicalisation'. More and more people, it is said, live in ways that hurt their bodies and put them at marginally increased risk for developing disease. If they are treated for this, they will never forget that they are really ill in some peculiar way, though still not ill, and they will be dependent on regular checks and many will experience side effects of the drugs. But, of course, some will also be prevented from developing premature organ failure, like cardiac failure, ischaemic heart disease or stroke.

GPs seem more reluctant than their more specialised colleagues – such as cardiologists or diabetologists – to follow this path of intensified search for health hazards. Possibly, the side effects of such ambitions become more visible in primary care, where physicians and nurses can hardly remain unaware of what happens when large parts of the population become 'pathologised' and put onto regimens of drug treatment. Possibly, we have here a source of mounting irritation between doctors with different tasks and different perspectives on health and illness.

An everyday example may illustrate the dilemma. The stress on risks has made a seemingly clear cut decision to check a person's blood lipids both scientifically and ethically complex and ambiguous. What may at first seem to be a wise line of action – to search for preventable risks for a patient – becomes a very delicate balancing of pros and cons. If, say, 140 patients with a certain constellation of parameters, the large majority of them asymptomatic, need to be treated with a drug in order that one of them may be prevented from having a stroke during a certain time period – then how shall we evaluate this scientifically and what would the ethical implications of such a line of action be?[12] How should we value potential side effects of drugs against their benefits? What will happen to persons when they are declared sick although they feel well, and how is this to be taken into account? How is their way of thinking about their bodies and their future affected? Are the costs for such large-scale projects acceptable?

We may conclude that looking for asymptomatic deviations and diagnosing them as risk factors may be very beneficial to some patients, but may in other cases be the opposite. Close knowledge of persons, a thorough but soundly critical knowledge of evidence-based medicine, a capacity to individualise and a keen eye for the larger socio-cultural aspects of declaring more and more healthy people as sick – these might help to ward off the most unwanted consequences of the spread of diagnoses.

BECOMING A DIAGNOSIS

Diagnosis sometimes cuts deeply into people's lives. Like most labelling it has a strong effect on thoughts and feelings and hence also on the sequence of events that will result from it. Diagnosis may in this way play the role of a self-fulfilling prophecy. The way we look at ourselves (as a 'diabetic' or 'psoriatic' or an 'epileptic'), and the way others look at us when we are given this label, will step by step transform us into something that we may not want to be. There are open or hidden expectations that strongly form those who carry such 'sickness roles', expectations that may be heavy to bear but not easily done away with. Hence, a diagnosis may strip a patient of his personality, of what is uniquely him, and replace it with stereotypical assumptions, hardly conscious for the one who holds them, of what it is to 'be' such a diagnosis. Yes, 'be' a diagnosis, because in this situation the diagnosis has taken on an existence of its own, has expanded far beyond the purposes for which it was constructed and become an obstacle to any attempt to restore the humanity of the ill. Thus, we still often talk of 'the brain tumour in room 4', or the 'schizophrenic' next door. Innocent as it may seem, it testifies to the inclination to reify individuals, to make them into their diagnoses.

ENIGMATIC SYNDROMES: FIGHTS OVER DIAGNOSES

Diagnostic 'battles' between patient and doctor would seem unlikely in the face of the enormous superiority in medical knowledge that the doctor possesses. This is, however, not the case and may be even less so in the future. When diagnosis is complex and uncertain, when the patient is discontented and does not feel relieved or helped, and when other diagnostic options open up (for example inspired by reading on the internet) – then it can happen that the patient does not accept what the physician suggests and chooses a different hypothesis, sometimes held with fervour and deep conviction. This alternative diagnosis might furthermore be supported by some other professional, a medically trained one or, perhaps, a representative of the huge field of CAM – complementary and alternative medicine.

Certain syndromes invite this predicament. What has been called 'enigmatic syndromes' offer challenges that are not always resolved in a constructive manner. 'Electricity hyper-sensitivity', to take one example, is a peculiar and in some ways also provocative situation, where a person experiences different unpleasant symptoms when exposed to very low-grade electro-magnetic fields. The general position of medical science is that these persons, who define themselves as 'allergic' to electricity, are 'psychologically' ill, that is that there is no organic pathology resulting from the exposure to such electrical fields. Blind tests in laboratories on some of these persons support this conjecture. But this does not prevent this group of patients from remaining firmly convinced about the aetiology of their ailment and taking the full consequences of it, for instance isolating themselves in small houses in the forest without any electrical devices at all.

This is an extreme and unusual example, but it illustrates a diagnostic dilemma in which doctors find themselves. What if there is no solid basis for medical diagnoses and what if the patient has strong ideas about her own disease? Should the physician accept diagnoses that are not scientifically plausible as 'healing myths'? Should one give in to the patient's wish for an explanation, for an ordering principle that gives a meaning to what goes on? If diagnosis means legitimacy, recognition and at least some sort of hope, who is the doctor to deny his patient such when he is incapable of offering anything better?

SUMMING UP

Diagnosis is an indispensable though not innocent way of labelling unwanted bodily and mental states. This is the essential paradox: diagnosis is both wanted and unwanted. Most of us would rather not be ill, but being ill without a diagnosis is usually worse than being ill with one. Diagnosis is the confirmation of the presence of unwanted disease and illness, but also a promise of a way out of it or at least to some relief.

Temperance and restraint might be more central virtues today than earlier. The technological options that might be triggered by a diagnosis are massive in the early 21st century. If diagnoses are to be used, they must be used with caution, sound judgement and restraint. The physician who is a good diagnostician not only knows many diagnoses, and is able to diagnose precisely – she also has the capacity to avoid diagnosis when diagnosis is futile and avoid labelling when labelling stigmatises. She will be able to handle diagnostic uncertainty when it appears, and knows that it will appear often. She will accept and handle the fundamental ambiguity of diagnosis: that it points to both an objective bodily dysfunction, but also and at the same time to an inner world where worry and uncertainty, hope and despair coexist. If the physician manages this, diagnosis will be the ill person's best friend.

REFERENCES

1 All contributions in some way or other illuminate this fact, but it is particularly dealt with in the last contribution, 'Giving meaning to symptoms'.
2 We see this tension appearing in the Middle Ages, where Aquinas considered human knowledge to be a knowledge of universals, where the particulars were instances of the existing universal categories. Ockham, in contrast, put an emphasis on human empirical knowledge as the creator of categories, suitable to individual cases. See Tarnas R. *The Passion of the Western Mind.* London: Pimlico; 1991, pp. 179–208.
3 If one still wants to use the verb, why not then say that we construct our interpretations (though that would perhaps also seem somewhat . . . yes, 'constructed'?)
4 Hellström O. The importance of a holistic concept of health for health care. Examples from the clinic. *Theoretical Medicine.* 1993; 14(4): 325–42.
5 Kathryn Montgomery notes this in her important book *How Doctors Think: Clinical Judgement and the Practice of Medicine.* Oxford: Oxford University Press; 2006. Alvan Feinstein makes the same observation with great clarity in his now classical book on *Clinical Judgment* from 1973.
6 Good B. *Medicine, Rationality, Experience: An Anthropological Perspective.* New York: Cambridge University Press; 1990, p. 78.
7 Evans M. The medical body as philosophy's arena. *Theoretical Medicine and Bioethics.* 2001; 22: 17–32.
8 Of course it should be noted that a lot of diagnosing is done by ill persons themselves, when for example ill with common colds, minor injuries or back pain. This 'lay man diagnosing' stands in an interesting and complicated mutual interplay with medical diagnoses, and is of great interest when physicians reach their diagnosis.
9 The VAS scale (Visual Analogue Scale) represents an attempt to quantify one of the experiences that is most difficult to quantify: pain. From very mild pain, 1, up to intense intractable pain, 10, the person with pain is asked to mark on a line where his own pain experience is.

10 Johannisson K. *Tecknen: Läkaren och konsten att läsa kroppar. (The Signs: The Physician and the Art of Reading Bodies)*. Stockholm: Norstedts; 2004, pp. 22–5.

11 Illich I. *Limits to Medicine. Medical Nemesis. The Expropriation of Health*. London: M Boyars; 1976.

12 In epidemiological literature, this average number of persons that need to be treated to prevent one disease incident is called NNT, Number Needed to Treat.

CHAPTER 3

Diagnosis: telling and hearing

JILL GORDON

One can argue that the end of diagnosis is not merely epistemic – what the physician has to know to institute the most appropriate treatment – nor is it always immediately directed to interventions and treatments to alleviate pain, suffering and, perhaps, to forestall death, but often, and more importantly, aims at the establishment of a trust relationship between patient and physician, which is critical to establishing the limits of the diagnostic process.[1]

He sat down close to me. 'I have bad news, I'm sorry. The tests are positive,' he said gently . . . Then I said the oddest thing – and I remember exactly the words because I caught myself choosing them carefully. 'I'm sorry,' I said, 'that it fell to you to tell me.' He looked a bit startled, but I meant it: at that moment I was struck by how unbearable it must be for him to sit beside people like this, week in and week out, and have to say what he'd just said to me . . . and then I was walking home again, barely connected to time and space, shrunken into the tiniest dot. I stopped at lights, crossed roads, passed blocks of flats, but I still wasn't there. From wherever I was, I just kept an eye on the moving dot, like an ant at the bottom of a pit.[2]

Robert Dessaix's *Night Letters* is a fictionalised account of his actual experience of HIV infection diagnosed in 1995, when HIV was still widely seen as a terminal illness. Dessaix describes the diagnosis as a terrible annunciation, from a doctor whom he describes as a 'Gabriel . . . Nor were his tidings a blessing. Nor did a dove glide down towards me on a golden beam – more a dry-mouthed raven with little yellow eyes on a bolt of black lightning.'[3]

In basic cellular terms the human immunodeficiency virus attacks and destroys cells in the immune system. In personal and relational terms, the diagnosis of HIV attacks and destroys the rich intricacy of an entire life, profoundly affecting one's self-concept, future expectations, and the attitudes of others.

> Crumpling, foundering, caving in, I kept one eye on the face across from me. The face was alertly serene in a way I knew, even at a moment like that, I liked. Plummeting, I fixed my eyes on his eyes, as if he were peering down into the well I was falling further into . . . the gentle questioning began and I tried to call back up to him, yet felt too crushed to speak.[4]

Dessaix's account suggests a clinical relationship that is close to ideal. He liked and trusted the doctor whose responsibility it was to deliver this terrible diagnosis. He found him 'alertly serene' – attentive but calm; when he needed to elicit more information, the doctor's tone was gentle.

We have already observed that causation can be viewed as a web rather than a single chain of events.[5] In the case of HIV infection the web involves the virus itself, the particular populations that are likely to be affected, the different moral status attributed, for example, to those who were infected by blood products rather than by sexual activity, the controversies surrounding public health campaigns, and many other elements; not only biological but moral, social and even political factors create the web. Each of them may influence the way in which the diagnosis is shared between doctor and patient, and the way the future of the clinical relationship is mapped out.

In Chapter 1, Rolf Ahlzén draws the distinction between the biomedical 'why?' and the existential 'why?' The correct biomedical diagnosis is unarguably important; the existential elements of the patient's predicament less arguably so. It all depends on what doctors are 'meant' to do. Doctors themselves are likely to view the onset of most diseases as arbitrary, carrying no special messages about our status as humans. Some patients would agree, treating their bodies as machines and their doctors as biomedical mechanics. This approach works well for relatively trivial diseases and injuries. However, the onset of serious illness does hold existential significance for all patients to a greater or lesser degree. We ask: 'Why me?', 'Why now?' 'What does this illness say about me?' 'How does it affect the way I see myself?' 'What has the meaning of my life been?' Should the doctor, sensing that these questions are forming, try to help the patient to address the existential questions, or expect the patient to manage alone, in a process that is quite separate from the medical consultation? – 'The test results show that you are HIV positive.' No more, no less.

When a patient is struggling to deal, as Dessaix was dealing, with a serious diagnosis, does the doctor have a moral obligation to try to alleviate the patient's sense of vulnerability and isolation? The answer seems obvious, on the grounds of sheer humanity alone, but not all doctors behave like Robert Dessaix's doctor. Even in the face of a life-threatening diagnosis, not all patients are shown such gentleness. Perhaps the origin of 'gentle' from the Latin *gentilis* 'of the same family or clan' suggests the reason for the difference; there are doctors who naturally perceive all of their patients as belonging to the same family or clan and doctors who do not feel such close affiliation (literally 'the adoption of a son'). The feeling of closeness or distance is related not only to personality, but also to cultural, social and other differences, as Iona Heath has described it in Chapter 5. The fact that doctors are often drawn from a different socio-economic background from their patients can increase the distance between them, and has been used to support the arguments in favour of widening access to medical education, in order to admit students from a wider variety of socio-economic backgrounds.

What kind of communication is best suited to the situation in which a patient who construes the diagnosis as having existential significance meets a doctor whose explanations are strictly biomedical? It may be that the patient needs to find a different doctor, to avoid an endless string of misunderstandings, but it may also be possible for the doctor to reconsider the limits of what s/he is offering as therapy. Perhaps the doctor could learn from the patient how the illness looks from his or her angle.[6] If such an effort can be made, then it may deepen the doctor's understanding of patients in general as well as leading to better health outcomes.

PERMISSION TO SPEAK

The central importance of the moment of diagnosis is underscored by the restrictions sometimes placed on the act, and the sanctions against unregistered persons who claim the right to offer diagnoses. In Ontario Canada, diagnosis comes under the Regulated Health Professions Act (RHPA) as a 'controlled act which may only be performed by professionals registered with either the College of Psychologists or the Royal College of Physicians and Surgeons'.[7] The professionals are doctors, dentists, psychologists, chiropractors, optometrists and podiatrists. Nurses, physiotherapists, occupational therapists and others are excluded. Such regulation raises significant questions about professional autonomy and power, and especially the tension that has existed and continues to exist in some respects between the professional roles of doctors and nurses.[8] At the heart of the question lies the right to give to, or withhold from another person, information concerning their health status. Many pages of regulation in countries across the world outline the limits of what nurses may tell patients. By contrast, there are relatively few legal constraints on doctors communicating diagnoses in medicine, even when doctors provide advice outside their particular specialty, or even engage in health scams.

THE PHYSICIAN AS PRIEST

In the past, diagnosis and healing have been seen as divine gifts possessed by individuals singled out for the role of priest or shaman. In some parts of the world, these beliefs continue. Although Western medicine has been remarkably successful in identifying biological links between disease and illness, mystical beliefs remain even in Western cultures. When patients' world views include, for example, the notion that their illness is part of some cosmic plan – that 'my number was up' or 'it was meant to be' – it is not surprising that they continue to link the role of the physician to the role of the priest.

The mixture of physicianly and priestly roles is inescapable. William Osler saw many priestly elements in the nature of the good physician. He speaks of imperturbability as one characteristic, which 'has the nature of a divine gift, a blessing to the possessor, a comfort to all who come in contact with him.'[9] Butler *et al.* have advanced the idea that the soteriological (or salvational) role is inescapable, because there will always be patients who use medical symptoms as a way of engaging their doctor with problems that are fundamentally existential.[10]

Since Osler's time the secularisation process has gathered even greater strength. Among the significant changes in medical education and clinical practice can be numbered the shift to a molecular rather than a whole person focus, the patient being regarded at times as an irritating appendage to an interesting pathological process. Even the proposed solutions, such as improved communications skills training for medical students, can be relentlessly reductionist in nature.

Fifty years ago, Szasz and Hollander addressed the question of medical authority and described three behavioural styles that physicians adopt.[11] They designated these as 'active-passive', 'guidance-cooperative' and 'mutual participation'. The active-passive relationship is characterised by the doctor's paternalism and the patient's unquestioning belief and dependency. With this style of interaction, the doctor maintains control over the information that is communicated, to whom it is communicated and when it is communicated.

With an increasingly well educated population with ready access to information, especially in the developed world, the active-passive relationship has become more difficult to sustain. While it still persists, especially among some older doctors, the profession has tended toward recognising the potential benefits of the more open communication styles of guidance-cooperation and mutual participation. In helping to define patient-centred medicine, Moira Stewart, among many others, emphasises the need for a balance between diagnosing disease and demonstrating understanding of the illness experience.[12,13]

In attempting to interpret the patient's illness and suffering, the doctor's role approximates the role of priest. From an historical and cross-cultural perspective, ethicist David Barnard has argued that 'modern Western medicine's insistence on a purely scientific and technical approach to healing, shorn of every vestige of mystery, faith and religion, is an aberration on the world scene. It appears as a detour, albeit with some indispensable achievements along the way, from humanity's common pathways in the confrontation with suffering.'[14]

There are innumerable opinions, and a large body of research concerning patients' preferences for receiving and dealing with medical information.[15,16] In the UK, the shift toward a 'patient-led' NHS does not leave much room for 'mystery, faith and religion'; its rhetoric is solidly focused on customers, outcomes and deliverables.[17] Similarly in the US, McNutt, for example, adopts a decidedly un-priestlike point of view in which the irritation is almost palpable:

> Some clinicians might think it is necessary to continue to share a patient's decision making, perhaps believing that doing so will make choices easer for the patient. However, no one should suggest that the goal of medical decision making is to make decisions making easy. On the contrary, the goal should be

to make it difficult; to make sure that patients understand that every decision is influenced by uncertainty and risk. The ideal is not to reduce decisional conflict, but to maximize it.[18]

Is this the kind of approach to communication that patients want? Robert Dessaix, in his time of crisis, wanted his doctor to take a more active, priestly role. Depending on the circumstances, patients may need their physician to adopt different styles – active-passive; guidance-cooperative, mutual participation and different patients may want different 'doses' of each style. When we consider 'our' patients – Rachel, Jake, Liz, Geoff and Jen – it seems clear that they want a doctor who communicates compassion and understanding along with the medical information that they need. They are in need of support and comfort. 'Maximising decisional discomfort' seems to miss entirely the points raised by ethicists such as David Barnard, who writes:

> Physicians are not priests. They have their own work to do. At the same time, their medical work has three aspects that make inevitable their assumption of some form of priestly role. First, the nature of illness is such that patients present themselves with existential – and not only biophysical – distress, and pin on the physician intense existential hopes. Second, the treatment relationship itself, with its demands on the physician's personal qualities of care and concern, is a critical mode of therapy. Third, medical work is value-laden in both its individual and social contexts.[19]

These three roles are clear in Dessaix's record of his experience. First, he is explicit in naming his doctor as 'Gabriel'. In the middle of a consultation about a deadly virus, Dessaix's naming reveals his own preoccupations, his perspectives and his cultural and religious essence. The diagnosis of a terrible disease lays bear his sexuality and the sexuality of the doctor, risks the doctor's disapproval but may also confirm his understanding. The 'annunciation' of his diagnosis has implications for the future, just as Mary, big with child, would become a subject of gossip and speculation, had Joseph not taken her as his wife. Dessaix may already be thinking about how this annunciation will be followed by the stigmata of facial lipoatrophy and skin changes that will inform both friends and strangers of his illness.

Barnard's second point is that the doctor communicates a diagnosis within a relationship that ought to be essentially therapeutic. Finally Barnard argues that medical work is value-laden in both its individual and social contexts.

The doctors treating Rachel, Jake, Liz, Geoff and Jen inevitably place a value on each of them, just as the patients will place a value on their doctors. One of the clearest manifestations of this valuing process is the amount of time that each provides for, or seeks from, the other.

Vanderpool and Levin see enduring links between medicine and religion.[20] Both medicine and religion place a high value on human life, seek to define and redefine ethical rights and wrongs, strive to alleviate suffering, try to help people to manage their lives better, and work to enhance our understanding of the human condition. In the process of conveying a diagnosis, the doctor encounters opportunities to do each of these things. Unless s/he is aware of, and committed to, these functions, the diagnosis may be limited by concern for its technical accuracy and its practical implications (decisions on therapy, further tests). This is not surprising, since these are the central themes of clinical education and training. A good clinical outcome is undoubtedly a central goal of medicine, but there are other important goals such as the relief of suffering, enhanced trust, a re-examination of personal priorities and new insights, as Dessaix's experience illustrates. Interweaving communication skills with ethical theory challenges students to develop their capacity for philosophical reasoning, a capacity that will contribute to decision making throughout their careers.[21]

THE PHYSICIAN AS 20TH CENTURY CULTURAL HERO

Physicians are still perceived as holding special knowledge and power, if television programmes from the 20th century are any guide. Myerhoff and Larson describe the medical doctor as a 'cultural hero'.[22] The hero functions to promote social integration in modern societies that lack a shared body of religious belief to provide ultimate sacred values.

This may help to explain the popularity of medical dramas and 'soaps' on television. Myerhoff and Larson's observations were contemporaneous with the enormously popular '60s TV soaps *Ben Casey* and *Dr Kildare*. Dr Ben Casey was portrayed as taciturn but competent, courageous and kind. Dr Kildare was younger, more sensitive and communicative, but equally astute in diagnosis. Both were unequivocal heroes, always concerned for their patients first and invariably coming up with the correct diagnosis. *Marcus Welby, MD* took over the public imagination in 1969 as a kindly but slightly unorthodox family doctor. That series was viewed by one in every four American households and in 1970 ranked number one among all TV series.

The change in the public perception of doctor-heroes began with the series *M*A*S*H*, inspired by a 1968 novel of the same name. The medical stars were Dr Hawkeye Pierce and Dr Trapper John McIntyre. The characters use resourceful good humour to cope in a mobile army surgical hospital during the Korean War. Both the producers and actors were amazed by the show's success, the final show in 1983 becoming the most watched episode in television history. Unlike *Ben Casey* and *Dr Kildare*, *MASH* was inspired by surgeons who actually worked in such an environment during the Korean War, their stories creating an influential anti-war statement. In taking such a line, the series also chose to represent the doctors as less purely heroic, quirkier people who defied or subverted authority, detested pomposity and hypocrisy and defended the underdog regardless of race or rank. Their communication with patients was humane and empathic in proportion to the humanity of the patients themselves.

In the 21st century, the heroes in *Grey's Anatomy*, *Cardiac Arrest* and *ER* demonstrate a variety of communication styles that move even further away from the uncomplicated, all-knowing hero. An ensemble of medicos take on different personae, some as bizarre as that of *House*, the eponymous hero of the Emmy award-winning American TV drama. Dr House is a brilliant diagnostician, but also a Vicodin-abusing eccentric, who ignores most of the rules of doctor-patient communication and whose misanthropic attitude toward patients has created his familiar by-words 'the patient is lying'.

The conditions covered by such series cover a wide spectrum of conditions from cancer to depression, brain damage, sexually transmitted infections, epilepsy, rape and drug addiction. Other anti-hero types in the UK include the star of the *Doc Martin* series, who blunders through the sleepy coastal village of Port Wenn. He is an excellent diagnostician, but his communication errors are unending and provide most of the material for each episode of the series. Jed Mercurio's doctor characters in *Cardiac Arrest* and *Bodies* are also heavily flawed, and there are abundant communication failures at all levels of the medical hierarchy. This remarkable change over a 40-year period is presumably a response to changing popular tastes and needs. If Myerhoff and Larson's view of the doctor as cultural hero is apt, then the period from the 1960s to the present day has seen the emergence of a much more complex and fallible figure, often quite inept in communicating with patients and colleagues and definitely not priestly by nature.

Is it possible that this decline in the mystery and power of the cultural hero reflects the reality of the medical world? Today, it is more likely that the person communicating a diagnosis to a patient will be female rather than male, and that regardless of sex, s/he may have a totally different cultural background from the patient. What was once a social and economic divide between wealthy, well educated male doctors and their poorer patients is now as likely to be related to sex, religion and cultural differences, and the doctors will not necessarily be part of the dominant group in any of these categories. The communication that occurs between patients and their doctors tends to be based on fewer assumptions about the doctor's superiority in status and power.

GETTING IT RIGHT

Communicating a serious diagnosis creates a unique moment in the consultation. Dessaix describes the immediate impact for him:

> It's a moment of such solitude, such nakedness, so utterly unlike any other, that we tend to look away from it politely as from an obscenity. If it is obscene it's because it leaves us shamelessly stripped of our learnt humanity, as animal, as instinctual as any monkey. Yet it's a moment that comes in the end to almost everyone.[23]

What Dessaix captures in these words is the loneliness of being singled out; the recognition, in existential terms, of our personal isolation, felt especially keenly in times of crisis. In everyday life, we prefer to forget these times – the nakedness, the stripping of our learnt humanity – that happen in a consulting room or hospital ward. Doctors are responsible not only for communicating a diagnosis, but for observing and working through its aftermath.

Recently I was speaking with a medical student who registered a particular sense of bewilderment and shock when he recounted how a consultant had communicated a serious diagnosis to a patient in a hospital bed, and then immediately answered his mobile phone which happened to ring at that moment. What amazed the student was the fact that the consultant continued the conversation with the caller for some minutes while the patient wept in front of him. When he finally ended the phone conversation, he did not acknowledge her emotional reaction to the news, but provided some technically oriented information and then left.

What Dessaix has described as 'a moment of such solitude, such nakedness' is bad enough by itself. When the doctor displays apparent indifference to suffering, the healing aspect of his or her role is not only lost, it is dangerously reversed, exacerbating the patient's pain and distress. The human element of the interaction cannot fail to have an influence – it unavoidably supports or damages the healing process. Such behaviour is not easily forgotten.

Patients also see the diagnostic process as something more than a moment of communication. Analysing narratives written by patients with cancer diagnoses, Salander found that:

> the participants often described experiences from the first contact with hospital staff to the end of their treatment, rather than as a single instance of diagnosis communication . . . From the perspective of the physicians, 'bad news' focuses on how to provide information about diagnosis and prognosis in the course of a single diagnostic consultation. From the patient's perspective, 'bad news' reflects the process of being diseased by cancer, and . . . in this relationship information about diagnosis and treatment is more a means than an end.[24]

Although there are various well-developed guidelines for conveying bad news, Eggly *et al.* point out that the process is not always so clear-cut in practice.[25] They identified three problem areas: one, that the moment of communicating a diagnosis may be difficult to plan, two, that the communication inevitably involves more than one item of information and, three, that the doctor-patient relationship is not the only relationship to consider – other professionals and family members almost always need to be included. The processes of communication that they observed were nonlinear, unscripted and highly complex. They recommend that, rather than relying on static communication guidelines, healthcare providers need to sustain a flexible response to patients' informational and emotional needs.

This helps to explain why doctors may instinctively equivocate over the delivery of a diagnosis. Instead of 'You have diabetes', one is more likely to hear the doctor say 'I think you may have diabetes' or 'diabetes is a possibility – we'll do a few more tests', making the delivery a staged procedure. An apparently simple word – diabetes, cancer, hypertension, depression – may have significant ethical as well as health implications. We know that patients cannot absorb information easily in the presence of bad news; it is generally understood that people need time. When Liz received the letter to tell her that her smear test was inadequate, the message did not actually hit home until the taxi taking her off on a holiday was almost at the airport. Jake too found it hard to concentrate on his GP's explanation after an unexpected intrusion into his body in the form of a rectal examination.

A policeman or emergency physician who must inform relatives of a sudden death may begin by stating that an accident has occurred, that the person was badly injured, that the paramedics/doctors tried to save them, but were unsuccessful, and finally that the person has died. Even if it only takes a minute to make these statements, it makes it possible to the listener's imagination to leap forward to the worst possible news, then back again, dreading, denying and bargaining, all in milliseconds. The compassionate doctor watches for evidence that the truth is being grasped before s/he makes a definitive statement that sets off the process of grieving for the life that existed just a moment ago; once that threshold has been crossed, both patient and doctor enter a different space.

When Dessaix realised that HIV/AIDS might be the explanation for his symptoms he recalled

> desperately wanting to drag time backwards just by a second or two, and rerun the scene with different dialogue, now, before it's too late: 'It looks like that flu that's going around . . . the wooziness, the lack of appetite . . . Take a few days off, I'll write you out a prescription . . .' Please say it again like that. Please.[26]

Rachel and her mother do not even know the doctor who delivers the diagnosis of diabetes; she is the youngest doctor in the ward, with her hair 'scruffed up in a clip at the back of her head'. There is no name associated with Rachel's doctor, she is simply one of the legion of tired, overworked and replaceable junior doctors marching through the hospital wards on their way to whatever future career lies ahead. Rachel's doctor has a pat formula, full of assumptions, for communicating with children of Rachel's age:

> 'You're a smart girl. It won't make you any different. You'll be able to do everything you want to do,' she said. 'Just like before. Being diabetic doesn't mean you have to change your dreams.'

The busy hospital leaves little scope for the doctor to match her pace, style and the content of communication with Rachel's needs for appropriately tailored information and reassurance. She has no idea of the extent to which the mention of injections tortures Rachel with visions of school nurses wielding large needles. In this situation, the diagnosis comes in the form of an informational 'package' backed up by the 'special diabetes nurse'. It is not the beginning of a therapeutic relationship – the doctor may never see Rachel again. It is a diagnosis given in the absence of a future responsibility.

TIME

Claude Debussy described music as the space between the notes, and in a medical consultation, the space between the items of information can be just as vital to the full composition that creates a consultation. Adequate time is an essential feature; Howie *et al.* and other researchers have validated its use as a proxy measure for overall quality of care in general practice.[27] No other single measure can do better.

Each of the doctors in our stories is 'time poor'. Julian Tudor Hart's inverse care law states that 'the availability of good medical care tends to vary inversely with the need of the population served. This inverse care law operates more completely where medical care is most exposed to market forces, and less so where such exposure is reduced.'[28] Doctors extend the inverse care law by spending more time explaining diagnoses to those who need it least.[29,30]

Time is not the only factor that may be lacking. Some doctors, and perhaps especially those with a strong biomedical focus, are not skilled in observing and interpreting the nuances of their own behaviour or the behaviour of others. They may choose to ignore the fact that patients have different needs based on different cultural, social or family norms. The mismatch between the socio-economic and social status of the doctor and his or her patients may also create a wide communication gulf between them. Failure to recognise, interpret or make allowances for these differences can be frustrating for both the doctor and the patient and dramatically reduce the therapeutic potential of the diagnostic moment. Unfortunately it may also increase the risk of diagnostic errors.

UNCERTAINTY AND REASSURANCE

How comforting to be the physician who, in Chaucer's Canterbury Tales,

> . . . knew the cause of every malady,
> If it was hot or cold or moist or dry
> And where its seat and what its composition:
> You'd nowhere find a more adept physician.
> And when he knew the cause of the disease
> He'd give the patient fitting remedies.

In Rachel's case the diagnosis is unequivocal and the doctor can speak with confidence. Jake, however, has a syndrome, a cluster of symptoms and/or signs that literally 'run together' without a clearly defined explanatory mechanism. They are an admission of medical uncertainty.

An uncertain diagnosis leaves both doctor and patient free to worry about all of the worst possibilities. Doctors sometimes try to reduce anxiety (in themselves and others) with words of reassurance, regardless of the likelihood that the ultimate diagnosis will point to a serious or benign condition. However, their behaviour may have the opposite effect. Rief *et al.* have shown that patients are likely to incorrectly recall the medical conditions that the doctor says they probably do *not* have, rather than the benign condition that they most probably do have.[31] The words describing diseases stick more firmly than the words describing non-diseases. In thinking about the right words to use, doctors also juggle other anxieties, such as fears of litigation, their own natural conservatism or their awareness of the adverse personal and social implications of a particular diagnosis. Doctors may therefore find themselves walking a fine line in communicating the concept of risk rather than moralising.

As well as dealing with uncertainty in diagnosis, doctors are also responsible for conveying information about elevated risk of disease. We now know more than ever about risk, based on epidemiological research. Increasingly, doctors are engaged in providing information about risk to a relatively healthy patient group, rather than information about disease. Doctors are being encouraged to be advocates for healthy lifestyles, but many of the habits that affect health in Western societies – alcohol use, inactivity and obesity for example – are also associated with both illness and social disapproval, because they are construed as representing weak will, sloth or self-indulgence.

The information to be communicated may be as precise and definitive as a diagnosis of HIV or diabetes, as elusive as irritable bowel syndrome, as vague and frightening as a shadow on a chest X-ray.

HOPE, TRUST AND TRUTH

A diagnosis of a significant medical condition changes the patient's self-concept. Thirty years ago, Haynes *et al.* showed that being diagnosed with hypertension can lead to increased absenteeism, even though the hypertension is itself asymptomatic.[32] A diagnosis can lead to loss of one's identity as a well person, loss of control, or loss of capacity and autonomy. On the other hand, the news of a diagnosis may also bring relief, when it offers an explanation for particular symptoms, and validates the patient's lived experience. A diagnosis, properly handled, is part of the therapy. Handled clumsily, it may simply add to the patient's overall burden. For Rachel, it is bad enough to know she has diabetes, but even worse to be told, by someone who knows little about her, 'You'll be able to do everything you want to do.' How could the doctor possibly know what Rachel wants to do?

Jake's busy GP, Dr Siddha, communicates the diagnosis is a way that overwhelms him with information:

> 'Your problems certainly tick all the boxes for IBS.'
>
> 'IBS.' Jake thought that sounded like a computer.
>
> 'Irritable Bowel Syndrome.' Dr Siddha clicked her mouse and the printer on her desk began to hum. 'Here,' she handed him the newly typed prescription, and a larger sheet of paper. 'Here's some information for you. Come back if these don't help, or if things get worse. Don't exceed the stated dose. Have you any questions?'

In the pressured world of general practice, it may be difficult to establish a trust relationship. The time pressure and lack of familiarity that threaten the trust relationship between Dr Siddha and Jake are also operating when Jen goes to the hospital clinic to see Dr Murray about a shadow on her chest X-ray.

> 'It's TB, is it Doctor?'
>
> The doctor shook his head. 'No, Not TB. That would be most unlikely . . .. A different sort of shadow. We need to do more tests, then work out a treatment plan. Cancer is a possibility.'

Kindly Dr Murray must communicate the diagnosis at some time, but he cannot be expected to know Jen as a person, or to understand her personal circumstances. Spicker observes:

> The failure of contemporary physicians to earn the honor of 'good physician' can be found in their attitudes toward the handicapped (or potentially handicapped) patients . . . a large number of diagnoses . . . unduly suggest physician failure. As a consequence, the physician is in danger of missing an extraordinary opportunity to focus on and attend positively to each patient's self integrity and integral self image . . . and thereby is far less likely to suggest strategies that may lead the patient to initiate the complex process of acceptance of an integrated new form of life . . .[33]

When our baby daughter was found to have a club foot many years ago, three orthopaedic surgeons were involved in her care. Over the first few years of her life she needed a number of surgical procedures. None of the doctors mentioned the practical implications of the condition, until a friend who happens to be an orthopaedic specialist, said simply 'She won't limp. She'll need to choose from a more limited range of school sports – swimming rather than running, for example. Her left calf will always be smaller than the right, so she may, in her teenage years, prefer wearing jeans to dresses.' Most important of all, he added 'oh, and you mustn't feel guilty when those stretching exercises you've been given don't bring her calf up to normal size. No amount of exercise will do that.'

Those were exactly the things we needed to know! How wonderfully welcome was all that information about day-to-day life as part of the 'package' of care that we needed. The surgical correction was only a tiny fraction of the picture, and yet, over and over, doctors ignore or brush over their patients' lived reality, the practical implications of each diagnosis. Between them, those specialists must have seen hundreds of children with talipes deformities. Even more intriguingly, they were themselves fathers and they were kind men.

Communicating that diagnosis was important for the whole family. Another diagnosis had a similar effect. The rapid onset of severe 'wet' macular degeneration came as a complete surprise to my mother in 2000. At 86 she was enjoying relatively good health and living independently in a small retirement unit. She knitted all the time and was a member of a small group that produced a huge number of knitted items to be donated to the Salvation Army every three months. She cooked a lot and often brought scones, small cakes and her special fruitcake when she came to visit.

When she became partially blind in the left eye, we began the rounds of ophthalmology consultations, confirmed the diagnosis and saw four different doctors for laser treatments of one kind or another. The disease progressed remorselessly and she made a tremendous effort not be overwhelmed by the sheer terror of it. The left eye lost all central vision and the vision in right eye began to deteriorate rapidly. I accompanied her to the consultations. The first and fourth doctors were kind but business-like, the second distant and technically oriented (when he realised that I was a doctor, his manner softened very slightly, a response that I find infuriating).

The third doctor was different. Half-way through the consultation she asked my mother about the things that gave her pleasure. 'I loved to read,' my mother said, and then added 'and TV, good films, plays and my knitting and my cooking'. The doctor touched my mother lightly on the forearm (I can see her hand as I write) and she said simply 'This is such a cruel disease.' No more, no less – in particular, no platitudes. Her voice tone left no doubt that she understood to the extent that any sighted person could possibly understand.

She continued with the consultation.

When we walked outside, my mother said 'Wasn't she a wonderful doctor?' I don't think she knew why she felt that way. Nothing else about the consultations was essentially different – the waiting rooms, the instructions, the drops, the slit lamps, the images on the TV monitors. All of the consultations took about the same amount of time. The retinal vessels kept on leaking and leaking, too diffuse for the laser treatment to stop, far less reverse, the damage. My mother's vision disappeared almost completely, but whenever the topic of her treatment came up, she would always mention, not the failure of the treatment, but that 'lovely doctor'. The 'lovely doctor' was simply doing what every doctor could do every day, without any additional time or technical expertise. If all doctors took such opportunities, the benefits to patients of the doctor's priestly power would be incalculable.

Hope has been defined as 'positive expectations for goal attainment'.[34] Because it arouses positive expectations, hope is associated with enhanced problem solving and motivation to succeed. Those are exactly the attributes that Rachel, Jake, Liz, Geoff and Jen need as they face the implications of their respective diagnoses. Eliott and Olver found in interviews with patients with terminal cancer that 'hope' can be construed as a noun that focuses on the probability of cure from a medical point of view ('there is no hope') or as a verb that emphasises the patient's active engagement in life and relationships with others, regardless of the medical facts of the case. It is a potentially damaging mistake for doctors to think only in terms of hope-as-a noun, that is, in purely biomedical terms. Even if a patient's hope has no impact on the progression of a disease, it is clearly valuable in itself.

Daniel Sokal argues that the duty to be honest with patients may, on rare occasions, be overridden by the desire to shield them from a grim diagnosis.[35] He offers two criteria for assessing whether deception can ever be justified: one is to ask whether one would be willing to defend the choice before a body of reasonable people (such as a committee of one's peers or a court of law). The second is to imagine the likelihood of the patient himself or herself consenting to the deception. Sokal suggests that a proxy measure of the latter criterion might be to ask the patient's relatives what they think his or her preferences might be. This is difficult territory, dangerously close to the unjustified paternalism from which the profession is still extracting itself. There are, however, occasions on which patients have said that they were glad not to have known about a serious diagnosis at a particular time in their lives.

Communicating a diagnosis is one of the most important moments in the doctor-patient relationship. David Thomasma sees healthcare as 'a personal healing activity, carried out through institutions that embody values such as respect for persons, the value of human life, and duties to care for individuals who suffer'. Healthcare systems that are poorly organised or under-resourced make it difficult for doctors to do it well.[36] Adhering to consultation guidelines laid down by the General Medical Council was shown to double the length of clinic consultations in otolaryngology, and it is likely that this finding is generalisable to other specialties.[37] Clinicians are left with a choice between adherence to GMC guidelines and meeting clinical need. If the basic conditions for good doctor-patient communication are not met by the healthcare system, then doctors deserve praise for managing the communication process as well as they do under the circumstances.

Robert Dessaix faced a diagnosis almost as terrifying as cancer. Another diagnosis with similar dread connotations is multiple sclerosis. A study of communication in the diagnosis of multiple sclerosis found that 'all patients reported the moment as powerfully evocative and unforgettable'.[38] All felt that the diagnosis could be made less painful if they were provided with an appropriate setting (privacy, no interruptions, sufficient time), tailored information and continuity of care. These two factors – the doctor-patient relationship and the structure and organisation of healthcare – are crucial to the success of the process.

Symptoms are always potentially serious. When we find out that they are trivial, we smile with relief and chide ourselves for worrying about nothing. When we find out that they are an indication of a serious illness, everything changes. We are reminded of the doctors' special role as intermediary, not between man and God, but between man and death.

> Doctors, after all, are almost the only people we allow to talk directly of death. It can't be pleasurable, but, like a small child, a doctor is given leave to sit and talk to you in detail about your dying, if not your being dead. In its way it's quite refreshing. Everyone else, you soon discover, whether sad, concerned, excited (and that does happen) or merely anxious that you go without leaving a mess behind you, tends to talk to you about everything else except death . . . (but) unless you consider it, how can you know how best to live now? Without

thinking through what death means to you, aren't you walking backwards towards a precipice? Much better, surely, to walk facing what's ahead, stepping forwards with care, judging your footing and pace.[39]

REFERENCES

1 Spicker S. Ethics in diagnosis. In: JPD Gracia, editor. *The Ethics of Diagnosis*. Dordrecht: Kluwer; 1992, p. 114.

2 Dessaix R. *Night Letters: A journey through Switzerland and Italy*. Sydney: Pan Macmillan; 1996; pp. 108–9.

3 Ibid., p. 5.

4 Ibid., p. 7.

5 Krieger N. Epidemiology and the web of causation: has anyone seen the spider? *Social Science & Medicine*. 1994; **39**: 887–903.

6 Tuckett D, Boulton M, Olson C, Williams A. *Meeting Between Experts: An approach to sharing ideas in medical consultations*. London: Tavistock Publications; 1985.

7 *Regulated Health Professions Act 1991*, SO 1991, c. 18. Ontario: Government of Ontario; 1991.

8 Fairman J. Delegated by default or negotiated by need? Physicians, nurse practitioners and the process of clinical thinking. In: E Baer, P D'Antonio, S Rinker, J Linaugh, editors. *Enduring Issues in American Nursing*. New York: Springer; 2000.

9 Osler W. *Aequanimitas: With Other Addresses to Medical Students, Nurses and Practitioners of Medicine*. London: HK Lewis; 1904, p. 4.

10 Butler CC, Evans M, Greaves D, Simpson S. Medically unexplained symptoms: the biopsychosocial model found wanting. *J R Soc Med*. 2004; **97**: 219–22.

11 Szasz T, Hollander M. A contribution to the philosophy of medicine and the basic models of the doctor patient relationship. *Arch Intern Med*. 1956; **9**: 585–92.

12 Stewart M. Effective physician-patient communication and health outcomes: a review. *Can Med Assoc J*. 1995; **152**: 1423–33.

13 Stewart M, Brown J, Donner A, McWhinney I, Oates J, Weston W *et al*. The impact of patient-centered care on outcomes. *J Fam Pract*. 2000; **49**: 796–804.

14 Barnard D. The physician as priest, revisited. *Journal of Religion and Health*. 1985; **24**: 272–86.

15 Arora N, McHorney C. Patient preferences for medical decision making: who really wants to participate? *Medical Care*. 2000; **38**: 335–41.

16 McNutt RA. Shared medical decision making: problems, process, progress. *JAMA*. 2004; **292**: 2516–18.

17 Department of Health. *Creating a Patient-led NHS – Delivering the NHS Improvement Plan*. London: Department of Health; 2005. Report No. ROCR Ref 4699.

18 McNutt, op. cit.

19 Barnard, op. cit., p. 284.

20 Vanderpool H, Levin J. Religion and medicine: how are they related? *Journal of Religion and Health*. 1990; **29**: 9–20.

21 Lamb D, Easton S. Philosophy of medicine in the United Kingdom. *Theoretical Medicine and Bioethics*. 1982; **3**: 3–34.

22 Myerhoff B, Larson W. The doctor as a culture hero: the routinization of charisma. *Human Organization*. 1965; **24**: 188–92.

23 Dessaix, op. cit., p. 6.

24 Salander P. Bad news from the patient's perspective: an analysis of the written narratives of newly diagnosed cancer patients. *Social Science & Medicine*. 2002; **55**: 721–32.

25 Eggly S, Penner L, Albrecht TL *et al*. Discussing bad news in the outpatient oncology clinic: rethinking current communication guidelines. *J Clin Oncol*. 2006; **24**: 716–19.

26 Dessaix, op.cit., p. 7.

27 Howie J, Heaney D, Maxwell M. Measuring quality in general practice: pilot study of needs, process and outcome measures. *J R Coll Gen Pract*. 1997; **75**: 1–32.

28 Tudor Hart J. The inverse care law. *The Lancet*. 1971; **297**: 405–12.

29 Smedley B, Stith A, Nelson A. *Unequal Treatment: Confronting Racial and Ethnic Disparities in Health Care*. Washington, DC: National Academy Press; 2002.

30 Furler JS, Harris E, Chondros P *et al*. The inverse care law revisited: impact of disadvantaged location on accessing longer GP consultation times. *Med J Aust*. 2002; **177**: 80–3.

31 Rief W, Heitmüller A, Reisberg K, Rüddel H. Why reassurance fails in patients with unexplained symptoms: an experimental investigation of remembered probabilities. *PLoS Med*. 2006; **3**.

32 Haynes R, Sackett D, Taylor D *et al*. Increased absenteeism from work after detection and labeling of hypertensive patients. *N Engl J Med*. 1978; **299**: 741–4.

33 Spicker, op. cit.

34 Eliott J, Olver I. Hope and hoping in the talk of dying cancer patients. *Social Science & Medicine*. 2007; **64**: 138–49.

35 Sokal D. Can deceiving patients be morally acceptable? *BMJ*. 2007; **334**: 984–6.

36 Thomasma D. The ethics of managed care: challenges to the principles of relationship-centered care. *J Allied Health*. 1996; **25**: 233–46.

37 Banerjee A, Yates PD, Hawthorne MR. The effect of GMC guidelines on the length of otolaryngological out-patient clinics in a district general hospital. *Clinical Otolaryngology*. 2002; **27**: 335–7.

38 Solari A, Acquarone N, Pucci E *et al*. Communicating the diagnosis of multiple sclerosis: a qualitative study. *Multiple Sclerosis*. 2007; **13**: 763–69.

39 Dessaix, op. cit., p. 111.

CHAPTER 4

The dialogue of the clinical encounter

RAIMO PUUSTINEN

DOCTORS AND PATIENTS

Middle East

The man walked in with his completely veiled wife. I couldn't even see her eyes. The woman stayed in the corner while the man sat down in front of me. He explained something in Arabic and the male interpreter translated it to me in broken English. It appeared that the woman was suffering from abdominal pains of some kind. I tried to inquire more deeply into the woman's problem but the husband refused to offer any more details. I urged the interpreter to ask the woman about her problem but he told me that it was not possible for him to address her directly. It also appeared that I was not allowed to perform a physical examination on her. I solved the problem by inviting a female physician together with female interpreter to take over. We three men left the room while the women stayed behind the closed doors to discuss the patient's problem.

Central Africa

The doctor introduced me to a young boy with newly diagnosed diabetes. He told me with his thick Indian accent how the boy had been carried by his mother from far away to this remote clinic near the Ugandan border. The boy had been severely dehydrated on arrival but he seemed to be quite alright now.

A young visiting internist from a world famous medical school in the US was making notes and asked the doctor how they controlled the patient's 24 hour blood sugar levels. The doctor smiled sadly when he said that they don't. They only have one kind of insulin anyway and when the boy leaves the clinic he is going to die since there is no way he can obtain continuous medication from where he lives. I said hello to the boy but he just stared at us quietly. There was no linen on the rusty hospital bed. The concrete walls were stained and flies were swarming around the boy's head. We went to the next bed where a man was dying from pulmonary tuberculosis. He was gasping for breath as we moved on.

Northern Europe

Two paramedics rushed through the main door pushing stretchers. There was blood all around. 'Male 45, car accident, severe injuries to the head, BP 100/60, P 120 . . .'

The ER nurse took notes while the paramedics were calling out the vital signs. The patient's face was lacerated and his eyes wandered around. He looked at me when I called him by his name. He uttered something before he passed out.

Eastern Finland

The lady was staring at the floor, sobbing. 'He was such a good boy. And now . . . I don't know what I have done wrong'. I was running late, and now this lady whose son had blown his head off with a shotgun the night before . . . I sat quietly, letting the lady cry. Three more patients waiting and I should be on my way in twenty minutes.

FRAMES AND AIMS

We physicians are often accused of not listening to our patients. We are told that we just read laboratory results, stare at our computers and ignore our patients as persons. This claim has been levelled at us for so long that is has created a whole new line of inquiry in medicine and on medicine. Piles of books and articles have been published on doctor-patient communication, and teaching communication skills has become commonplace in many if not most medical schools throughout the world.

I am not convinced that we physicians are as poor communicators as a species as one may assume on the grounds of all this academic activity. Instead, I would like to claim that on the whole we doctors do listen to our patients and we listen carefully. The question might rather be: what do we actually listen to when we listen to our patients?

Our task as physicians is to understand the workings and frailties of the human body and mind and to find ways to cure and alleviate the problems our patients present to us. To give a simple example: If the patient approaches a physician and complains that there is blood coming from the rectum, our task is to find out exactly where that blood comes from, why is it coming, stop the bleeding and to prevent it from happening again. In order to succeed we need to start our inquiry by listening to what the patient tells us about his or her symptoms. When we listen, we try to discern bits and pieces of information that may help us to decide on the likely nature of the underlying cause for the bleeding. That is to say, we concentrate on what we consider relevant to solve the problem the patient presents as his or her reason for consulting us at that particular moment.

Yet the patients do not automatically disclose all the relevant information. This is why we need to ask questions of our patients, to gain a fuller picture of what is going on in their bodies and minds. We may also need to know where, how and with whom that particular patient lives and what s/he does or does not do for a living. These queries cannot, however, be presented as a set of preformulated questions in the hope of gaining complete and rational answers from our patients. Instead, they need to be formulated and adjusted anew for each and every consultation and its aims.

For example, in a busy Emergency Department the task is to concentrate on immediately life-threatening issues. That limits the scope of communication to the questions relevant for the objectives of the ED. There is not much point in engaging in a discussion of the patient's marital problems or traumatic childhood memories, when the patient is blue and breathless and we don't know why. The communication skill needed is to ask the right questions and ask them quickly. This is why many emigrating physicians prefer to work in emergency departments and in anaesthesia when working in an alien language environment. It is easier to learn to say in any language 'where does it hurt?', 'open your mouth', 'have a deep breath' than to master the language to the full, as needed to be able to practise as, say, a general practitioner or a psychiatrist.

Furthermore, to give another example of the influence of context on the mode of doctor-patient communication: when I was working in Saudi Arabia as a GP it was virtually impossible for me to discuss with my female patients any of their problems occurring between their navel and knees and, in many cases, in any part of the body. If I managed to get an idea about what was going on through the accompanying male relative and a local interpreter, it was categorically impossible for me to perform a pelvic examination for my female patients even in cases of acute vaginal bleeding. This could be performed by female physicians only. It is quite obvious that there would be no possibility of approaching my female patients in that particular culture, no matter how many courses I took to improve my communication skills

Finally, if one works in a remote makeshift clinic somewhere in Africa, seeing daily a hundred patients who speak a variety of local dialects and having only paracetamol, penicillin, quinine and basic surgery as one's therapeutic arsenal, one does not get involved in discussing the finer points of each and every patient's symptoms or their personal problems. On the other hand, one needs to develop a very special type of communication skills to be able to make sound clinical judgements in those circumstances.

This is not to say, however, that we should not take the issue of the clinical dialogue seriously. On the contrary, it is a more serious issue than we often think. That is to say, proper communication with one's patient is not only a matter of good manners and patient satisfaction. The dialogue between the patient and the physician is, in effect, the most important aspect of medical examination and treatment. After all, most of our clinical encounters take place in non-hurried circumstances with patients who are not critically ill. The patient is talking and the doctor is listening. The patient's problem is unfolding through the dialogue that takes place, guiding the doctor toward a diagnosis and treatment. But how does this actually happen, usually in a matter of a few minutes?

THE OPENING

When the patient approaches a physician s/he has a problem s/he has considered as in need of a medical consultation. Except in emergency situations the patient has usually prepared an opening presentation. When the physician asks why the patient has come to the surgery the patient says, for example, that his or her shoulder has been aching for some time. That opening sentence orients the physician's thinking to follow a certain line of reasoning, which is different if the patient says that s/he is feeling tired all the time. Whatever the patient utters as his or her opening statement leads the physician to set off on the path of reasoning that s/he has adopted through training and experience for that particular type of problem. One may compare it to a drop-down menu on a computer screen. Press 'aching shoulder' and you get a different menu then when pressing 'tired all the time'. However, the similarities with computing do not go any further than that. Doctor-patient communication does not follow rigid problem-solving algorithms, as we shall see, and this is the reason why the attempts to build clinically reliable computer-based diagnostic programs have not fulfilled the expectations, at least as yet.[1]

The patient expresses in his or her opening statement what s/he considers as relevant to explain his or her reason for seeing the physician. S/he is thus, as Osler once remarked, giving the diagnosis, at least to the point of giving it a working title: 'Aching shoulder'; 'Tired all the time'. The patient's opening presentation is, however, insufficient, vague and perhaps completely wrong from a diagnostic point of view. After all, this is precisely the reason why s/he is seeing the physician. S/he is there to gain better understanding of and/or to find an explanation, cure or alleviation for his or her problem.

Since the patient's opening statement usually discloses the information the patient holds as relevant to his or her problem, interrupting that statement is not just bad manners but plain stupid, because it is the most valuable tool for the physician to make progress. This is why all the textbooks of medicine underline that the patient should be given sufficient time to present his or her case uninterrupted. Studies published on the length of the patients' opening statements show that in most the cases they spend less than a minute in telling the physician the reason for the visit.[2] Even if the opening speech takes longer than that, it is time well spent since it provides more information and, if nothing more, time to observe the patient. And if the patient keeps on talking for ten minutes or so – which is extremely rare in any case – the physician may wonder whether it is a sign of a mental disorder worthy of further exploration.

By the time the patient finishes the opening statement the physician has a drop-down menu, or several menus, open. S/he has also observed the patient's physical appearance, state of mind and emotional status and related all this to his or her previous knowledge of the patient, if there is any. But during the few opening moments of the consultation the patient has done precisely the same. How does the doctor look? Does s/he seem interested in me? Busy? Friendly? Detached? Frightening? Trustworthy? Indeed, can I trust this physician? Does s/he know what s/he is doing? S/he looks so young. S/he does not seem to listen to what I say. S/he is just staring at the computer screen.

PATIENT'S HISTORY

When the patient has completed an opening statement s/he waits for the physician's response. This moment is, perhaps, the most crucial of the medical examination. The physician has his or her menus open, but where to go from there?

It seldom, if ever, happens that the physician is able to 'close' the case on the basis of the patient's opening presentation. That may occur, for example, when a young woman who has urinary infections three times a year comes to see her physician and says 'here we go again'. Even then, the physician is not content to be a vending machine and to deliver the prescription wordlessly. S/he observes the patient and engages in a communication of some kind, even a short one, to make sure s/he understands the patient's complaint properly and does not miss a case of chlamydia, for instance. In most cases the physician needs to gain more information than the patient has presented in his or her opening statement. This is why the physician starts to ask questions. S/he starts, as we tend to say, to take the patient's history.

I would like to call into question here, however, the notion of a physician taking the patient's history. That is, I question that there exists such an entity as the patient's history just waiting to be 'taken' and analysed in an objective manner.

First of all, the patient is not an object of inquiry producing full answers to standard questions. The way the physician behaves affects the way the patient presents the opening statement and how s/he responds to the physician's questions and vice versa. That is why the clinical dialogue necessarily varies in words, intonations and gestures and consequently in the way the session proceeds. And this is precisely the reason why the computer analogy does not apply in a medical consultation, since the patient's and the physician's reactions to each other's utterances and behaviour in a living dialogue cannot be anticipated as a predetermined set of responses.

Furthermore, when the physician listens to the patient's opening presentation s/he is not hearing a factual statement as s/he might when a radiologist reports that there is a 2 cm stone in the patient's gall bladder. Instead, the physician is listening to the patient's subjective account of the problem that has brought him or her to the surgery. The way the patient expresses the problem is modified not only by his or her general ability to express symptoms and worries, but also by the language and dialect used, by the local ideas of illness and cure and, as we saw earlier, by the setting of the consultation, that is, whether s/he is talking to an unknown physician in a busy emergency clinic or to the local GP in the tranquillity of the familiar consultation room.

The notion 'taking the patient's history' is relevant, however, in the sense that patients do have a history. Their symptoms have persisted for some time, sometimes even months or years before they decide to come and see a doctor. 'Taking the patient's history' means, therefore, to construct what has happened before the patient's arrival at the surgery. In this sense a physician works as an historian attempting to find out what has happened before.

Physicians' training consists of a broad spread of natural sciences, accompanied by a side dish of social sciences and psychology and spiced with a hint of humanities. Due to our basic orientation to the human body as natural scientists, or biologists to be more exact, we tend to think of our patients' bodies as objects of inquiry. History to a physician is thus natural history, as when examining the development of an embryo, growth of a tumour or development of cardiac infarction during the critical ischaemic moments of coronary thrombosis. The problem is that when we inquire into our *patient's* history we are not observing specimens in a laboratory. We are conversing with living agents of our own kind.

The problem for a physician in clinical dialogue is that, if we fail to ask relevant questions, we may never get relevant information. And even when we do ask the right questions, we cannot be sure whether the answers we get are valid. Every seasoned clinician can tell endless stories concerning this problem. 'It never crossed my mind that this sweet old lady was an alcoholic when I was trying to figure out why she was getting dizzy every now and then, and having these bruises everywhere. I did ask her about alcohol once but she only smiled and said she would never touch a glass. Well, she must have been drinking straight from the bottle.'

The patient's history cannot, therefore, be taken as an object in its own right. It is, instead, mutually constructed between the physician and the patient during the consultation. To illustrate my argument, let us take a brief look at how professional historians reflect their trade.

The British historian E.H. Carr questioned in his famous Trevelyan lectures, delivered half a century ago, the idea of history as merely collecting the facts and reconstructing the past 'as it was'. He discussed the problem of obtaining facts in historical research by writing how 'the (historical) facts are really not at all like fish on the fishmonger's slab. They are like fish swimming about in a vast and sometimes inaccessible ocean; and what the historian catches will depend, partly on chance, but mainly on what part of the ocean he chooses to fish in and what tackle he chooses to use – the two factors being, of course, determined by the kind of fish he wants to catch. By and large, the historian will get the kind of facts he wants. History means interpretation.'[3] Therefore, for Carr, 'history . . . is a process of selection in terms of historical significance . . . history is a selective system not only of cognitive, but of causal, orientations to reality. Just as from the infinite ocean of facts the historian selects those which are significant for his purpose, so from the multiplicity of sequences of cause and effect he extracts those, and only those, which are historically significant; and the standard of historical significance is his ability to fit them into his pattern of rational explanation and interpretation. Other sequences of cause and effect have to be rejected as accidental, not because the relation between cause and effect is different, but because sequence itself is irrelevant.[4] . . . What, then, do we mean when we praise a historian for being objective, or say that one historian is more objective than another? Not, it is clear, simply that he gets his facts right, but rather that he chooses the right facts, or, in other words, that he applies the right standard of significance.'[5]

If we were to replace the words 'historian' and 'history' with the words 'physician' and 'medicine' in the quotations above, those paragraphs could be, curiously enough, an extract from any textbook of medicine discussing the problem of taking the patient's history. John Vincent writes in a similar vein in his recent book on the problem of evidence in historiography. Creating historical evidence is not, for Vincent, merely collecting facts. It is also about 'hunches, imagination, interpretation, guesswork. First and foremost, though, comes evidence: no evidence, no history.' But, for a historian, history 'is about intrinsically fallible evidence. In this it resembles medicine and the detection of crime. And it is about fallible evidence as interpreted by fallible people.'[6]

Vincent could be describing the medical consultation also when he notes that 'if history is about asking good questions, the evidence will not in itself choose what the questions ought to be . . . Two men digging in the same trench would produce different answers, because they were asking different questions.'[7] This phenomenon is familiar for physicians and patients alike. If a patient were to see different physicians with same complaints s/he would most likely end up having more or less different conversations and therapeutic suggestions with the physicians even when all reach the same diagnosis.

Vincent writes how 'history is about evidence, but only about evidence we approve of. Evidence we disapprove of, might as well not exist. We decide, even before looking at it, what can be evidence and what not.'[8] This observation also applies in medicine. To illustrate this with a clinical example, let us consider an elderly patient I treated in the Arabian Peninsula who pondered whether he was feeling ill because of the effects of an evil eye. Because in his community 'evil eye' is an everyday etiological possibility for various ailments, I considered the patient's expression as an indigenous metaphor holding no clinical evidence whatsoever. But if a deeply Lutheran bank manager in my hometown Tampere in Finland were to disclose to me that the pain in his tongue must be due to the evil eye cast on him by the mailman, I would consider that statement to be evidence not of tongue pathology but of psychiatric illness.

To conclude, in the medical consultation a physician faces the same epistemological problems as an historian who is interviewing participants in some event of historical interest and who is trying to construct what it was that took place and why in that particular period of time. In his introduction to modern historiography Michael Bentley says in summary that the past does not, by definition, exist. Therefore, it can never be reconstructed but only constructed in our present as a picture or image or model of the event of interest under our investigation.[9]

For the physician the material for diagnostic and therapeutic reasoning is created through the dialogue with the patient here and now. That is, the patient's history is constructed between the doctor and the patient in the always unique event of a medical consultation. The task a physician faces, when deliberating on the material that emerges during the clinical dialogue, is to decide what is relevant and what is not in terms of current medical theory and the aim of the consultation.

TWO LANGUAGES

In a medical consultation a doctor is conversing with one or more persons. Even when the patient is not able to talk (small child, paralysed, unconscious) someone has taken the patient to the surgery or hospital. The question of the conduct of the medical consultation is, therefore, also a question about the use of language and this is why linguists and socio-linguists have taken a central role in studying doctor-patient dialogue as a special form of human communication.

The language with which we converse in our ordinary encounters is not exact, fixed and final but it is open to all kinds of expressions and interpretations, as we can see in our everyday misunderstandings and quarrels. Scientific language, in contrast, attempts to be precise in its concepts and expressions. In the medical consultation ordinary language and scientific language meet. One of the doctor's many dilemmas is how to translate the patient's everyday language into medical concepts and how to create mutual understanding between medical thinking and the patient's comprehension of what is going on.

The way we express ourselves has developed through continuous interaction with other people. Our speech is thus moulded not only by our individual traits and capacities but also by the time and place we live in and people with whom we live. This is not just a matter of adopting a local language, dialect and style but also of content. The ideas we have about health and illness vary among our local traditions. Today these variations are perhaps greater than ever due to the all-encompassing media and to the commercial exploitation of a great variety of ideas and suggestions on illness and healing.

Physicians are also subjected to all of this. Despite the fact that the medicine we practise is based on scientific ideals and research, we have absorbed ways of thinking and expressing our thoughts from our own culture and immediate surroundings, long before we entered medical schools. Yet we like to think that since medicine is based on science, doctors are free from cultural assumptions and peculiarities. However, it is easy to see that when one goes from one country to another one finds different medical ideas and practices. Furthermore, this is not only the case between different countries, but also within any single country. One only needs to go from one clinic to another to find different practices. And finally, this phenomenon is not apparent just between different clinics but also between physicians within the same clinic. All of us physicians have our own ways of talking with our patients. One likes to have a thorough discussion with his or her patients while the other is rather quiet and asks only a few short questions.

However, despite of all this variability in the way we deal with our patients, we do not simply make a haphazard guess, or toss a coin, or plead for supernatural powers when we establish a diagnosis and prescribe a treatment. Instead, we apply scientific methods in the way we think and practise. That is, we rely on the scientific ideas we have about the structure, workings and malfunctions of a human body and mind as gained through our training. These ideas are expressed in scientific language as written in medical textbooks and journals and as spoken on medical congresses, meetings and bedside consultations.

This creates a certain tension in all doctor-patient encounters. We start with the patient's opening statement on his or her reason for attending the surgery. The physician responds to the patient's opening statement which leads to a discussion and conclusion of a certain kind. This dialogue is carried out in local language and dialect, coloured with the patient's expressions, ideas, fears and hopes and steered by the physician's responses, questions and answers. During the consultation the doctor's task is to translate the patient's expression into medical language leading to a diagnosis or, at least, to a plausible hypothesis on what might be going on, expressed in medical terms. In this process two languages meet, that of a layperson and that of medicine, which offers a set of possible ways the patient may or may not be considered as ill in a medical sense.

POLYPHONY AND MONOLOGUE

The tension between the patient's expression and the medical language can be seen, to use Russian linguist Mikhail Bakhtin's concepts, as the tension between the polyphony of everyday speech and the monologue of scientific language (Bakhtin 1996, 1997).[10,11] For Bakhtin the way we speak has been developed through continuous interaction with others and our expressions are, therefore, permeated with the voices of those with whom we have been associated. Indeed, we are able to notice in our speech phrases, intonations, opinions and ideas acquired from our parents, spouses, teachers, friends and associates. Every medical student (including myself long ago) has had as his or her hero a senior consultant during clinical training. One finds oneself not only clumsily using the terms and intonations the senior was using, but even imitating his or her mannerisms.

As a counterpoint to our everyday speech, medical textbooks and journals attempt to formalise the language we use, since in order to be scientific an expression cannot have multiple and contradictory meanings. A 2 cm stone in a gall bladder is a 2 cm stone in a gall bladder. A broken collar bone is a broken collar bone. Type A beta haemolytic streptococci in one's throat are type A beta haemolytic streptococci in one's throat. In the attempt to eradicate multiple meanings in their expressions the exact sciences constitute, in Bakhtin's terms, a monologic form of knowledge.

A physician needs to operate with and oscillate between these two modes of expression; the polyphony of everyday life and the monologue of medical language. And it is precisely along this axis that misunderstandings and dissatisfaction between patients and physicians present themselves. While a physician may be correct in medical diagnosis s/he may not notice within the patient's polyphony (approaching sometimes a cacophony) those aspects that are crucial for the patient. 'She did not listen to me,' complains the patient.

On the other hand, if the physician fails to establish a correct diagnosis, the patient may complain: 'He just kept asking these questions about my life while I had this tumour in my breast all the time.'

The tension between the polyphony of the patients' utterances and the monologue of medical terms can be vividly seen in our patient narratives. In our first story a young doctor is having a chat with Rachel, a teenage girl with newly diagnosed diabetes. The doctor explains the nature of her condition and how to treat it and tells her that she can live a normal life despite her disease. We are all assured that from a medical point of view that there is nothing to worry about. The condition can and will be treated. For Rachel this triggers a storm in her mind. 'Of course it worried me . . . so frightened of injections . . . all I could see in my head was that nurse's needle . . . I'm a *diabetic*? The word rang in my head like a hard, cold bell.' And when she encountered her family, the relationships were altered too. 'I could feel an ocean of worry in her . . . I've never known Mum to sit so still . . . I did not know what to do with her.'

The young physician addressing Rachel talked to her, not with her. The physician's position was monologic. She was not entering into a dialogue with the patient. A young, inexperienced physician in a busy hospital ward, tired from all that she has to manage, had a chat with – or to? – the patient and went on with her duties.

Jake, in turn, is visiting his local GP. He is ashamed of his condition with uncontrolled bowel movements and frightened by the appearance of blood in his stools. When he enters the physician's consultation room he enters the medical world. In his case the medical reasoning process requires a rectal examination. Jake isn't used to displaying his body and, what's even worse, the examination is about to be performed by a female physician. The doctor acknowledges the patient's embarrassment and does her best to cause the patient as little discomfort as possible. She keeps on talking while sliding the proctoscope into the anus. The doctor reassures the patient by saying there is nothing to worry about. Just piles, an everyday minor problem. She then explains the medical options and gives Jake some written instructions on how to deal with his bowel condition. The doctor pauses and offers the patient a chance to ask questions. Jake refuses; he has had enough for one day. The doctor then asks about his psoriasis. Jake is on his way out, just wishing to get away. He has used his six minutes and he does not crave for more. He has had a brief encounter with the monologue of medical diagnosis and treatment for IBS. Case closed. Reopening it is left to the patient.

In Liz's case the medical monologue is taken to the extreme. In the midst of her everyday haste comes a letter. A dry and factual statement about the need to take further smear tests since the previous test showed some minor abnormalities. Medical monology intrudes on the patient's life, triggering a whole symphony of questions, worries and fears. What is going on? Infection? VD? Cancer? Indeed, could it be cancer? Liz cannot concentrate, her hands are shaking, she feels sick. Damocles's sword hangs over her head. She desperately needs to hear a human voice to counter the monology of the letter.

She calls her physician, who instantly understands the patient's overwhelming worry. The doctor attempts to fit the demand of medical logic into the patient's life context. There is no need for her to worry; she should enjoy her holiday and have a day off when she comes back for re-testing, it is easier for her that way. The patient agrees and ends the call. She is shaking with relief.

In our fourth and final story the plot gets more complicated. Geoff has had a stroke. There is a permanent damage in his brain. From a curative perspective, the case is closed. The question is, however, how to offer him proper care while his wife, Jen, is tackling her lung problem.

For Jen the situation is dreadful. There is a shadow on her chest X-ray. From the medical point of view the challenge is to identify the nature of the biological process in her lung tissue causing the anomaly in the picture. For Jen the details of the cellular structure are of secondary importance. For her it is The Shadow In Her Chest X-Ray. For Jen the monologic medical expression is a matter of life and death. There comes to the surface the polyphonic story of her life. Her mother died because of a shadow. Her brother had it and became thin and stooped as he went through the agonising treatments.

The medical monologue begins again: Not likely TB though. Cancer, perhaps. An interesting diagnostic problem for a physician, to be solved with scientific methods. For Jen it is so much more than that. There are feelings of guilt because she knew she should not have smoked. And how to deal with her husband if she gets gravely ill? How to tell those closest to her what is going on? She is feeling sick, not because of the cellular process in her lungs but because she does not know how to incorporate all that into her life, for whatever time there is left to live.

Meanwhile, the doctor is assessing Jen's husband's condition. The medical monologue falls short: 'depressed', 'dehydrated'. What is needed, however, is not more medical terms but simply a means of taking care of him. The doctor tries to explain the situation to the patient but the patient is not listening. He is just staring at the wall. How can the doctor enter into a dialogue with this patient? What more should he say?

WHAT CAN ONE SAY?

Let us go back to the beginning, to the first moments of a medical consulta-tion. The patient has concluded the opening statement. The physician has the pull-down menus open. How should s/he proceed from here? What reply should s/he make? What question should s/he ask? Since each and every doctor-patient encounter is inevitably unique, there are no standard answers available. No clinical guidelines can tell us what to say. No laboratory readings can steer us here.

Whatever the physician says will lead the dialogue in one direction or another. Yet the consultation is not a one-way logical process. There are always returns, loops and dead ends. During the clinical dialogue both participants respond to each other's questions, answers, gestures and tone in a constant interplay. That is why a medical consultation cannot be cast into a preformu-lated script or notation. It is rather a moment of improvisation for a duet. Theme and variations. The patient sets the tune, key and tempo. The doctor joins in where the patient pauses and develops the theme further for the patient to continue. The dialogue brings forth new tones, accents and contrasts to proceed if all goes well to a harmonious cadence; that is, to a mutual under-standing of what the patient's problem is all about and what should and could be done for it. This is the jazz of medicine. But should no mutual understand-ing emerge, the consultation falls out of tune and ends up at its worst as mere noise, where the participants are not even able to share the same key.

So, as doctors we converse as best we can. We express ideas and opinions derived from our training and experience and from an understanding of human life in general, entering into a living dialogue with the patient. That dialogue may help us to arrive at a diagnosis and treatment and it may help the patient to feel that his or her plea has been heard and answered. What more can, or should, a physician achieve during the few fleeting moments of dialogue in an everyday clinical encounter?

NOTE ON MEDICAL HUMANITIES

The core function of medicine is the consultation. The patient's problem is defined through the dialogue between patient and physician. This dialogue is shaped and modified by various personal, cultural and linguistic factors. Examining the nature of the clinical dialogue clearly demonstrates the need for the humanities, drawing as one must on linguistics, semiotics, historiography, anthropology and more.

REFERENCES

1 Kawamoto K, Houlihan C, Balas E, Lobach D. Improving clinical practice using clinical decision support systems: a systematic review of trials to identify features critical to success. *BMJ.* 2005; **330**: 765.

2 Rabinowitz I, Luzzati R, Tamir A, Reis S. Length of patient's monologue, rate of completion, and relation to other components of the clinical encounter: observational intervention study in primary care. *BMJ.* 2004; **328**: 501–2.

3 Carr E. *What is History.* St Ives: Penguin Books; 1990, p. 23.

4 Ibid., p. 105.

5 Ibid., p. 123.

6 Vincent J. *History.* London: Continuum; 2005, p. 9.

7 Ibid., p. 42.

8 Ibid., p. 28.

9 Bentley M. *Modern Historiography. An Introduction.* Norfolk: Routledge; 2006, p. 21.

10 Bakhtin M. *Speech Genres and Other Late Essays.* Austin: University of Texas Press; 1996, p. 161.

11 Bakhtin M. *Problems of Dostoyevsky's Poetics.* Minneapolis: University of Minnesota Press; 1997.

CHAPTER 5

The double face of diagnosis

IONA HEATH

Diagnosis is the door to medicine and so it should not be surprising that there is much to learn from Janus, the Roman God of doorways and beginnings, whose two heads face in opposite directions.

January, the beginning of each new year, is named for Janus. Between 4 and 16 AD, Ovid wrote Fasti, his poetic exploration of the Roman Calendar, and in Book One he describes Janus:

> Two-headed Janus, source of the silently gliding year,
> The only god who is able to see behind him[1]

This capacity to face in two directions, to integrate two perspectives, is fundamental to diagnosis and this chapter explores the multiple double faces of diagnosis. However, throughout, it is perhaps well to remember that facing in two directions simultaneously is the attribute of a god which humans will struggle to achieve. Such is the challenge and fascination of diagnosis.

THE DOORWAY BETWEEN PAST AND FUTURE

The process of diagnosis assesses past events and present state and then uses these to predict a future. The patient provides an account of the beginnings of illness which stretches back into that patient's past life story to a distance which varies from minutes to decades. Through observation and the rituals of clinical examination, the doctor assesses the present state of the patient's body and mind. Then, if and when the doctor offers the patient a diagnostic label, or imposes one, a crucial transition occurs. The patient's story passes, as it were, through a doorway and makes a new beginning. This is because a diagnosis implies knowledge, however limited, of prognosis – of what will happen to the patient in the future, of how the diagnosed disease will affect the life of the patient. Diagnosis is informed by and, in turn, informs time.

> When a physician diagnoses a human's condition as illness, he changes the man's behavior by diagnosis: a social state has been added to a biophysical state by assigning the meaning of illness to disease. It is in this sense that a physician creates illness just as a lawmaker creates crime.[2]

As soon as Rachel is given her diagnosis of diabetes, she is told that 'from now on' she will have to take care of herself. A diagnosis changes the future – sometimes dramatically and irreversibly, sometimes almost imperceptibly. The effect of the change depends not only on the scientific knowledge of the diagnosed disease and its medical prognosis but on the symbolic and emotional importance of the diagnosis for the particular patient. This will depend crucially on the experiences of others close to the patient who have been given the same diagnostic label. Rachel's mum is terrified by the diagnosis of diabetes because she already has some knowledge of its implications. Rachel herself has a much more open and innocent approach to the diagnosis because she has, as yet, no direct personal experience of what it means. Jen's particular life experience means that the diagnosis of TB seems to hold even more terrors than that of cancer. Jake is completely bewildered by his diagnosis of Irritable Bowel Syndrome because he has no way of grasping it and is given no real opportunity to understand the nature of the condition that he is being offered. Since knowledge and fears of particular diseases are buried deep within family and cultural traditions and context, the information provided by the doctor at the time of diagnosis can make a crucial difference to the patient's experience of that diagnosis and the future it brings. Here it is instructive to note the difference between the care of Jake and Liz. Jake's doctor does what she is supposed to do and gives him written information about his diagnosis but she shows none of the empathic imagination of Liz's doctor which is used first to sense and then to snuff out her fear and panic.

THE DOORWAY BETWEEN THE PARTICULAR AND THE GENERAL

The experience of illness is necessarily lonely. The symptoms and sensations of illness are always particular to the individual subjected to them and modulated by the particular context of life story and situation. No-one else can experience another's symptom directly. The doctor approaches the patient's symptoms through deliberate use of the imagination and the skills of bodily empathy (see Chapter 8) and then sifts his or her understanding of the particular experience through the mesh of the scientific knowledge which has attempted to group the whole of human experience of illness into a taxonomy of disease. The doctor shares this task of linking the particular to the general with the poet who is engaged in transforming private feelings into words which are effectively the taxonomy of language.

Seamus Heaney gave his second book of poems the title *Door into the Dark* and later he described this as a gesture towards:

> this idea of poetry as a point of entry into the buried life of the feelings or as a point of exit for it. Words themselves are doors; Janus is to a certain extent their deity, looking back to a ramification of roots and associations and forward to a clarification of sense and meaning.[3]

This seems precisely the task of the doctor and the purpose of diagnosis: to look back to a ramification of roots and associations and forward to a clarification of sense and meaning. As we see from our stories, the tragedy is that while diagnosis almost always leads to a clarification of sense and meaning for the doctor, this clarification is rarely made so accessible to the patient. Nonetheless the fundamental task of the doctor is to locate sense and meaning and then share it with the patient.

Heaney has also likened the creation of poetry to fishing and again there are useful parallels for doctors.

> – in the writing of any poem, there's usually a line being cast from the circumference of your whole understanding towards intuitions and images down there in the memory pool. If you're lucky, you feel life moving at the other end of the line; the remembered thing starts off a chain reaction of words and associations, and at that moment what you need is the whole of your acquired knowledge and understanding, your cultural memory and literary awareness. You need them to come to your aid and throw a shape that will match and make sense of your excitement.[4]

The whole of the doctor's acquired knowledge, understanding, awareness, memory and experience (both personal and professional) are needed for each diagnostic task. The good doctor, like the good poet, never loses that sense of excitement.

William Carlos Williams was both poet and doctor and understood this well:

> My business, aside from the mere physical diagnosis, is to make a different sort of diagnosis concerning them as individuals, quite apart from anything for which they seek my advice. That fascinates me. From the very beginning that fascinated me even more than I myself knew.[5]

And the anthropologist Clifford Geertz again concurs with Heaney by emphasising the breadth and depth that must underpin effective diagnostic skills.

> – the reach of our minds, the range of signs we can manage somehow to interpret, is what defines the intellectual, emotional and moral space within which we live.[6]

And within which we work as doctors. In the stories, we see how Liz's doctor understands exactly what it is to be terrified by a simple single word of six letters and how that understanding is fundamental to what she is able to offer to her patient. We must hope that Rachel's special diabetic nurse will have similar skills.

THE DOORWAY BETWEEN BIOMEDICINE AND MORALITY

Many of the intractable problems of the diagnostic process relate to the enormous diversity of sorts of definition that are included in the classification of diseases used in Western medicine. Some have a firm foundation in biomedical science; others seem more in the nature of normative statements of social and moral acceptability. Rachel's diagnosis of type 1 diabetes mellitus and Jake's psoriasis have a robust basis in scientific knowledge of the anatomy, physiology and biochemistry of the disease process. This knowledge is matched by a clear understanding of the range and benefits of treatments that have the capacity to both extend and enhance life. On the other hand, Jake's Irritable Bowel Syndrome is an attempt to explain symptoms on the basis of disordered function but with no clearly identified pathology and Geoff's depression is a description of the doctor's perception of the patient's state of mind with no proven relation to either anatomy or physiology. Yet doctors have a tendency to apply these various sorts of diagnosis as if they all had the same validity and implied the same certainties and the same level of understanding.[7]

Alvan Feinstein has pointed out that during the 19th century and most of the 20th, taxonomy was the crucially important intellectual activity in medical science responsible for huge advances in the understanding of histopathology, pathology and pathophysiology. As a result, the taxonomy of pathophysiology has been an essential component of the reasoning and judgement used in good clinical practice. However, over the past 30 years, computer-mediated statistical diagnostic methods have linked symptoms and signs to pathological anatomy and bypassed detailed pathophysiological understanding.

> The incomplete clinical reasoning is encouraged by the silence of clinicians who know better, but whose innumeracy makes them insecure or intimidated when confronted by statistics.[8]

This use of statistics has discouraged further efforts at pathophysiological classification and the identification of potentially significant subgroups within existing categories. Many diagnostic categories remain huge baggy concepts whose clinical manifestations are extremely diverse.

Less hampered by the rigorous application of statistical methods in randomised controlled trials, psychiatric diagnostic classifications have developed in the opposite direction. In 1917 the American Psychiatric Association recognised 59 psychiatric disorders. With the introduction of the Diagnostic and Statistical Manual, the DSM, in 1952 this rose to 128. The second edition in 1968 had 159, the third in 1980 227, and the revision of the third (DSM-III-R) in 1987 had 253. Now we have DSM-IV, which has 347 categories.[9] This expansion represents not only extensive subdivision of existing categories but also broadening of the range of abnormality so that feelings and behaviours which were previously regarded as falling within the normal range of human experience of distress or eccentricity have now been reclassified as psychiatric disease. What does the huge expansion imply? Does it really represent the progress of science? Is the degree and extent of definition helpful to those who are ill or does it merely provide intellectual exercise for researchers?

> Even the most liberal system of psychiatric nomenclature does violence to the being of another. If we relate to people believing that we can categorize them,

we will neither identify or nurture the parts, the vital parts, of the other that transcends category. The enabling relationship always assumes that the other is never fully knowable.[10]

Patients and general practitioners can perhaps be forgiven some scepticism about the nature of psychiatric diagnosis. Anyone reading through the medical records of a patient with a chronic and enduring mental illness will notice the tendency for the diagnosis to shift over time. I have many patients whose mental condition has seemed largely unchanged but whose diagnosis has varied along an apparent continuum, which includes schizo-affective disorder, psychotic depression, borderline personality disorder and schizophrenia. The remarkable thing is how consistent the suggested treatments have been in the face of the changing diagnosis. The cynical view is that the diagnosis seems to matter little as the treatment options are few and are nearly always permutated until a relatively stable, but more or less satisfactory, outcome is achieved.

Many people feel increasingly uncomfortable about a substantial proportion of psychiatric diagnoses and the continuing history of the abuse of psychiatry as an instrument of political control casts a long shadow. Psychiatry describes deviations from a norm which is socially rather than scientifically defined. Science is too often used as a gloss to disguise the exercise of political power. The story of the inclusion of homosexuality within the DSM is very instructive. Homosexuality was not removed from the list of psychiatric diagnoses included in the DSM until 1973 and then only after sustained protests by gay activists. Both its original inclusion and its removal as a result of political protest demonstrate clearly the social construction of psychiatric diagnosis.

This social construction is most evident in mental illness but is by no means confined there.

> The medical act combines technical and moral decision making in a way which makes it a moral enterprise of a special kind. Each medical decision involves the complicated interplay of several value sets – those of the physician, of the patient, and of society.[11]

This situation is complicated and challenging even when the values of the doctor, the patient and their society are relatively concordant, but become proportionately more so when those values diverge.

– the word 'disease' has an evaluative character. Using it can be justified, if patients and doctors evaluate it in the same way – if patients agree with their doctors that the disease is bad for them. But it becomes problematic when this agreement is absent.[12]

THE DOORWAY BETWEEN ASYLUM AND STIGMA

To some extent every diagnosis brings both asylum and stigma. The proportions vary enormously but the doctor needs to be aware of the implications of both.

The conferring of a diagnostic label, even if it has serous implications, can bring enormous relief. Before diagnosis, many patients are bewildered and frightened with little understanding of what is happening to them and imagining a huge range of more or less terrifying possibilities. Both Rachel and her mother are relieved to find that there is a coherent explanation of what has happened to her and that treatment is available to relieve her distressing symptoms. It is possible that Jen's imminent diagnosis of cancer and not TB will come as a relief and Liz's fears are immediately relieved by the dismissal of the possibility that she most feared. On the other hand, Jake seems to find his diagnostic label much less useful and it is also conveyed by the doctor with much less conviction. Geoff seems almost oblivious to his diagnosis and, again, one wonders whether the label itself offers any additional benefit.

> – it may not be particularly helpful to think about depression as a specific medical condition . . . It encapsulates certain aspects of human experience, and in so doing sets artificial boundaries around them, conferring on them both the rights and responsibilities of an illness, and leading us towards treatment paradigms which tend to reduce – rather than enhance – our ability to live our lives.[13]

However, for many people a formal diagnosis of depression can provide a real sense of asylum – shelter from a maelstrom of feelings of, for example, regret, remorse, guilt or failure.

As soon as the patient has a diagnosis, there is the possibility of feeling less lonely because a diagnosis is necessarily a generalisation and implies the existence of a group of others who have been given the same label and with whom there should be at least the possibility of holding some experiences of illness in common. A diagnosis also gives access to healthcare professionals who have recognised expertise in that particular disease as happens to Rachel with the appearance of her diabetic nurse Dax. Fear and feelings can be shared and the diagnosis brings with it some idea of prognosis, albeit little more than a statistical prediction[14] with no guaranteed validity for any particular individual. In these ways, the patient immediately has more of an idea of the future but it is seldom enough, in the face of serious diagnosis, to vanquish fear completely. Rachel can still feel 'an ocean of worry' in her mum and needs to understand soon where that comes from and whether she will be obliged to share it or not.

A formal medical diagnosis legitimates a person's invalid status and excuses the inability to participate fully in family, work or community life. However, this always comes at a considerable personal price both in terms of suffering and of becoming trapped within the constraints of an externally imposed story. A diagnosis, particularly perhaps a mental illness diagnosis, seems to generate a momentum of its own, which can further undermine the patient's autonomy and capacity for self-realisation.

> The WHO definition of health as 'complete physical, social, and psychological well-being' says something that we must acknowledge: it is about a person's potential for living, which is a matter of autonomy and 'personal space', of having room to make choices. These are the concerns of general practice because our professional objectives are wider than the diagnosis and treatment of disease, but we too need to be careful lest diagnostic or therapeutic exuberance in the individual case blind us to our patients' needs for space and stature.[15]

These dangers should remind doctors always to remember Carl Edvard Rudebeck's injunction that:

> The most important motive for the confirmation of a diagnosis is practical, which means that the diagnosis never needs to be more accurate than what benefits the patient.[16]

This becomes particularly important in the face of the many diagnoses which carry obvious potential for stigma and it is interesting to note that those diagnoses which have a firm foundation in biomedical science are usually seen as much more 'respectable' and are much less likely to be stigmatising than those which have a more socially normative or moral basis. Liz might well feel that her epilepsy does not follow this pattern and there are many diseases, including epilepsy, which historically have been thought of as expressing moral failing but which are now, thankfully, rather better understood. Stigma, however, can be very persistent.

There is a socio-economic gradient for the prevalence of almost every major disease and these gradients are often steepest for psychiatric diseases.[17] The fourfold difference in the rates of male suicide between social classes I and V provides just one example. Again, questions arise about the point at which psychiatry becomes an agent of social control and, beyond that, a tool of political repression? As noted above, the history of psychiatry demonstrates that it is peculiarly susceptible to the medicalisation of political, socio-economic, racial and homophobic oppression – the medicalisation of 'otherness'. The discontent of the socio-economically deprived will always have the capacity to drive social unrest. But if the discontented can be described as depressed or found to be suffering from psychological distress, then they can be treated with pharmaceuticals or offered counselling. Social unrest is averted, the discontent is subverted and the injustices of society remain untouched. Nothing disturbs the comfortable complacency of those on the gaining side of injustice.

The borderline between humane care and social control is ill-defined and troubling. Those struggling to retain their dignity and to cope at the bottom of a steep socio-economic gradient are marginalised, and excluded from many of the conventional rewards of life. This exclusion may well be reflected in a rejection of 'normal' mainstream attitudes, priorities and behaviours, and, at the extreme of this process, behaviours come to be regarded as either mad or bad by the rest of society. There is constant need to guard against the tendency towards a rigid normalisation that exists within psychiatry, particularly when it is accompanied by insidious processes of stigmatisation. And these difficulties are further compounded by issues of cultural diversity and the differing understanding of different behaviours in different cultural contexts.

The doctor holds a gift of asylum within the diagnostic label but needs always to remember that he or she may also be conferring stigma. Perceptions of the stigma of each condition will be dependent on cultural and family traditions and need to be elicited if they are to be confronted. Some people may feel a condition to be powerfully stigmatising when those around them have no such sense. Jake's psoriasis may be just such a condition.

THE DOORWAY BETWEEN HEALTH AND RISK

Current enthusiasm for extending longevity and preventing disease through the identification of risk has added a whole new dimension to the challenge and complexity of the diagnostic process. As David Sackett has emphasised, therapeutic medicine and preventive medicine have completely different moral foundations.

> The two disciplines [of curative and preventive medicine] are absolutely and fundamentally different in their obligations and implied promises to the individuals whose lives they modify.[18]

When someone feels unwell and seeks relief of symptoms, the doctor has a clear responsibility to do his or her best but cannot guarantee success. In primary preventive care, the doctor seeks out the patient rather than vice versa and, with an implicit promise of benefit, offers someone who is at present in good health an intervention which is expected to make their life better in the future. Unfortunately, all such interventions oblige the recipient to consider a range of possible threats to their health and are almost always associated with a degree of heightened anxiety and fear. For some people, as began to happen with Liz, this fear can become overwhelming and debilitating in itself. In Denis Pereira Gray's memorable image, preventive interventions stain the clear water of health with the ink of fear and once stained the water can never be clear again.[19] Fear cannot be taken back. The diagnosis of risk is not something to be undertaken lightly or unthinkingly.

Unfortunately, the almost universal fear of death and the desire for longer and healthier lives is reflected in huge enthusiasm for preventive medicine on the part of government, the media, the public and some doctors. This enthusiasm is assiduously cultivated by the pharmaceutical and health technology industries and is driving the identification of more and more risk factors and more and more possible interventions for each of these.[20] An ever greater proportion of the population is being diagnosed as being at increased risk of serious disease or premature death, while most populations in rich countries are in fact living longer than ever before. Regrettably, very few people seem to be aware of the uncertainty of the connection between risk and actual disease in any particular individual, even for a risk factor as powerful as smoking. To what extent is the deliberate inflation of fear to drive participation in screening programmes justified and how well does the screening system either identify or accommodate the genuine preferences of individual patients? The role of screening in older people may simply be to change the cause of death rather than to prolong life.[21]

Clearly, the most significant threats to the lives and health of those who have yet to reach the average expectation of life should be identified and if possible minimised but risk thresholds that label three quarters of any population[22] as being at increased risk of premature death are clearly absurd and, by making the population more fearful, do more harm than good.

> For a human being is the creature who can think the future and who seeks to know how things will be in advance. But this distinguishing characteristic of human beings is also what makes them dangerous even to themselves.[23]

THE DOORWAY BETWEEN LOCKING IN AND OPENING OUT

Not all illness is caused by disease. A headache can be caused just as readily by suppressed anger or worry as it can by migraine or a brain tumour. When symptoms are caused by the disappointments, injustices and simple strains of daily life, there is little to be gained from recasting them as diseases. When that happens – or in the attempt to make it happen – patients are often subjected to unnecessary investigations which may in themselves be harmful. Further, a diagnostic label, once conferred, is very difficult to remove completely. The patient becomes locked into the diagnosis and all its implications.

At least 25% of symptoms presenting to general practice do not correlate with a recognised biomedical disease and it is important not to attempt to impose a diagnosis in this situation. If the symptoms of illness can be interpreted as, in some way, a reaction to the life circumstances of the particular patient, as is almost certainly the case with Jake's gastrointestinal problems, then, instead of being locked into a label, a whole range of different ways of resolving the problem will open out.

> Good general diagnosticians are rare, not because most doctors lack medical knowledge, but because most are incapable of taking in all the possibly relevant facts – emotional, historical, environmental as well as physical. They are searching for specific conditions instead of the truth about a man which may then suggest various conditions.[24]

The stated aspiration of general practitioners is to achieve a triple diagnosis which accommodates biological, psychological and social factors in an integrated assessment of a unique individual. If the patient is locked in too soon to a biological diagnosis very important psychological and social factors may be neglected. Dr Murray may be unable to see beyond Jen's cancer while Dr Siddha does not want to look beyond Jake's convenient label of Irritable Bowel Syndrome.

> Triple diagnoses change the nature of diagnosis from a label to a narrative which is full and moves through time.[25]

Even when a patient must be locked into a diagnosis, it is essential to open out the label to accommodate the particular patient so that, effectively, each disease becomes unique.

> When a diagnosis lands in a person, a new disease arises every time. Every time a new disease arises, sculptured by this person's unique history, character and life situation. Thereby, each person becomes ill in his own way.[26]

Each unique disease instantiates the general diagnostic label in the particular existential circumstances of the individual patient and, faced with this new disease, the task of both doctor and patient is to explore what it means within that particular patient's bodily person and life story. The aim is to re-establish sufficient equilibrium, within both the body and the narrative, to allow the patient's life to open out again.

> – health depends on many different factors and the final goal is not so much regaining health itself as enabling patients once again to enjoy the role they had previously fulfilled in their everyday lives.[27]

Technical medical treatment attempts to re-establish the equilibrium of the body. At the same time, conversation between patient and doctor has the capacity to restore the thread of a life story, disrupted by illness, because of the power of words to locate sense and meaning within experience even when that experience involves pain and suffering. Both processes are essential and both must be tailored to the state and circumstances of the individual.

Every *making of a diagnosis* is a profound commentary upon both the general scope of an abstract idea and the characteristics of an individual person. Janus faces in two directions simultaneously; doors allow movement both in and out. The challenge for the doctor on the threshold of all these doorways is to attempt always to look both ways at the same time. We aspire to see the past and the future, the particular and the general, the biomedical and the moral, possibilities of asylum and stigma, health and the risks to it – all simultaneously. We seek to follow Janus: we are not gods and so we fail but the aspiration is nonetheless essential.

Again, William Carlos Williams, doctor and poet, knew this:

> – in general it is the rest, the peace of mind that comes from adopting the patient's condition as one's own to be struggled with toward a solution during those minutes or that hour or those trying days when we are searching for causes, trying to relate this to that to build a reasonable basis for action which really gives us our peace.[28]

REFERENCES

1 Ovid. *Fasti Book I*. Translated by AS Kline. www.tonykline.co.uk/PITBR/Latin/Ovid FastiBkOne.htm (accessed 15 August 2007).

2 Freidson E. *Profession of Medicine: a study of the sociology of applied knowledge*. New York: Harper & Row; 1970, p. 223.

3 Heaney S. *Preoccupations: Selected Prose 1968–1978*. London: Faber and Faber; 1980, p. 52.

4 Heaney S. Lux perpetua. *The Guardian Review*. June 16 2001 (reprint from Poetry Book Society Bulletin).

5 Williams W. *The Doctor Stories*. New York: New Directions Books; 1984, p. 121.

6 Geertz C. *Available Light – Anthropological reflections on philosophical topics*. Princeton, NJ: Princeton University Press; 2000.

7 Malterud K, Hollnagel H. The magic influence of classification systems in clinical practice. *Scand J Prim Health Care*. 1997; **15**: 5–6.

8 Feinstein AR. The problem of cogent subgroups: a clinicostatistical tragedy. *J Clin Epidemiol*. 1998; **51**: 297–9.

9 Wessely S. The medicalisation of distress. *RSA Journal*. 1998; 4: 79–85.

10 Yalom I. *Love's Executioner and Other Tales of Psychotherapy*. Harmondsworth: Penguin Books; 1991.

11 Pellegrino E. Towards a reconstruction of medical morality: the primacy of the act of profession and the fact of illness. *Journal of Medicine and Philosophy*. 1979; 4: 32–56.

12 Boyd KM. Disease, illness, sickness, health, healing and wholeness: exploring some elusive concepts. *J Med Ethics: Medical Humanities*. 2000; **26**: 9–17.

13 Dowrick C. *Beyond Depression: a new approach to understanding and management*. Oxford: Oxford University Press; 2004: 5.

14 Nessa J, Malterud K. 'Feeling your large intestines a bit bound': clinical interaction – talk and gaze. *Scand J Prim Health Care*. 1998; **16**: 211–15.

15 Metcalfe D. The crucible. *J Roy Coll Gen Pract*. 1986; **36**: 349–54.

16 Rudebeck C-E. General practice and the dialogue of clinical practice: on symptoms, symptom presentations and bodily empathy. *Scand J Prim Health Care.* 1992; **Suppl 1**.

17 Thornicroft G. Social deprivation and rates of treated mental disorder: developing statistical models to predict psychiatric service utilisation. *British Journal of Psychiatry.* 1991; **158**: 475–84.

18 Sackett D. The arrogance of preventive medicine. *CMAJ.* 2002; **16**(4): 363–4.

19 Gray D. Evidence based medicine and patient centred medicine: the need to harmonise. *J Health Serv Res Policy.* 2005; **10**: 66–8.

20 McKinlay J, Marceau L. A tale of 3 tails. *American Journal of Public Health.* 1999; **89**: 295–8.

21 Mangin D, Sweeney K, Heath I. Preventive health care in elderly people needs rethinking. *BMJ.* 2007; **335**: 285–7.

22 Getz L, Kirkengen A, Hetlevik *et al.* Ethical dilemmas arising from implementation of the European guidelines on cardiovascular disease prevention in clinical practice. *Scand J Prim Health Care.* 2004; **22**: 202–8.

23 Gadamer H-G. *The Enigma of Health. The art of healing in a scientific age.* Stanford, CA: Stanford University Press; 1996, p. 85.

24 Berger J, Mohr J. *A Fortunate Man.* Harmondsworth: The Penguin Press; 1967, p. 73.

25 Pendleton D. www.edgecumbehealth.com/pdf/values_college_gp.pdf (accessed 13 December 2009).

26 Fugelli P. Trust – in general practice. *Br J Gen Pract.* 2001; **51**: 575–9.

27 Gadamer H-G, op. cit., p. 129.

28 Williams W, op. cit., p. 120.

CHAPTER 6

What do diagnoses mean, and does it matter?

PEKKA LOUHIALA

Very probably you have had *pharyngitis* at least once in your lifetime. If you are old enough, you may have *hypertension* or at least you know someone who has. More and more people in the Western world, like Rachel in one of the opening narratives of this volume, develop *diabetes*. But almost certainly you have not had *fourth disease* and definitely not *drapetomania*.

The words in italics are medical *diagnoses*. The first one is simply sore throat and the second one is high blood pressure, which is not a disease but may lead to, for example, stroke (the diagnosis Geoff had in another opening narrative). The third diagnosis implies a variety of symptoms and findings related to abnormal glucose tolerance. Fourth disease as a diagnosis was described in the late 19th century when childhood exanthemata were classified ('first disease' was measles, 'second disease' scarlet fever and 'third disease' rubella).[1] Its existence as a separate entity was controversial from the beginning and by the latter part of the 20th century it had been dropped from the medical textbooks. Arguments for the existence of fourth disease have been, however, presented as late as 2001.[2] Drapetomania was the tendency of black slaves to flee from captivity.

Pharyngitis, hypertension and diabetes as diagnoses are commonly used today but fourth disease and drapetomania have not been used by physicians for a long time. The diagnosis fourth disease bears no particular moral connotations but the very idea of drapetomania as a medical diagnosis sounds strange and morally appalling to us.

In the medical context, the concept *diagnosis* (Gr. *dia-* between/by, *gnosis* knowledge) refers both to the process of identifying a disease and also to the conclusion of the process. Much of the discussion below would be similar if the original question concerned *diseases*.

Medical knowledge changes rapidly and diagnoses are not an exception to this. Diagnoses come and go, and many factors outside medicine have an influence on their popularity. A broken bone is a broken bone anywhere and at any time but the prevalence of, e.g., *fibromyalgia* or *chronic fatigue syndrome* is highly dependent on cultural factors.

An impressive text about the cultural factors that shape the diagnosis and treatment of diseases is Lynn Payer's *Medicine & Culture*.[3,4] Payer lived and worked as a journalist in Britain, France, West Germany and the United States for several years and integrated personal experiences and extensive research into a fascinating book. This demonstrates elegantly how medical care depends upon some basic assumptions about the body and disease which are not based on scientific research. Two examples are the diagnoses *spasmophilia*, which was found only in France and *low blood pressure* which was actively treated in Germany but hardly ever in Britain. Since the publication of the book in 1988, many of the examples given by Payer are now out of date. However, differences surely remain and her message has not been weakened.

What is considered as a valid medical diagnosis and what is not may have major consequences in people's lives. In addition to medical consequences, there may be social consequences (e.g., in the case of alcoholism) or economic ones (e.g., if a particular condition is a valid cause for early retirement). A notable example is homosexuality, which during a short time changed from being regarded as a sin to a crime, then to a disease and finally to a normal variation of sexual behaviour.[5]

The universe of diagnoses seems to be expanding with the process of *medicalisation*. This refers to the expansion of the sphere of medicine by defining more and more previously non-medical issues and problems as medical ones. For example, menopausal symptoms, infertility or hyperactivity were not medical diagnoses just a few decades ago. Although medicalisation is often considered to be a negative phenomenon, it has also had positive consequences, for example in the elderly population. Effective treatments for cataract, hearing impairments, and osteoarthritis are good examples of such consequences.[6]

The term 'medicalisation' was introduced in 1972 by Irving Zola. During the past three decades medicalisation has received widespread attention among sociologists of medicine in particular. While the early critics of medicalisation focused on the role of the medical profession, the picture is more complex today.[7] The roles of modern biotechnology, consumers and managed care have become dominant and the role of doctors more subordinate in the expansion or contraction of medicalisation.

Recently, Nicolas Rose has pointed out that medicalisation as a phenomenon is much older than the term. Since at least the 18th century, medicine has played a part in 'making us what we are'.[8]

Rose distinguishes three dimensions of this process. First, our physical appearance, height, weight and longevity have been changed by developments in infrastructure, which are only partly medically controlled. Examples include sewage systems, purified water and food, dietary advice and the general sanitisation of human existence. Second, medicine is intertwined with the ways in which we experience and give meaning to our world. Through medical themes in literature, art, film and television, our imagination has become permeated with medicine; medical metaphors even inform theories of society. For example, we commonly refer to 'sick economies' or 'healthy societies'. Third, at least from the beginning of the 19th century medicine has had a role in governing the ways we conduct our lives. According to Rose, doctors have a good claim to be the first social scientists.

In the following, first, a typology of diagnoses is briefly described. Second, two classical philosophical problems, the problems of *universals* and *natural kinds* and their connection to the status of diagnoses are discussed. Third, value questions related to the formulation of diagnoses are examined. Fourth, as a conclusion, the relevance of all this from the patient's point of view is considered.

TYPOLOGY OF DIAGNOSES

It may not be possible to give a precise definition of diagnosis. Dictionaries and philosophers of medicine have given different definitions which emphasise various aspects. However, physicians make diagnoses all the time. Sometimes the diagnosis is obvious at first sight; sometimes the process is long and complicated. Very often there is a degree of uncertainty in the diagnosis, and sometimes no diagnosis at all is reached.

There are many classifications of diagnoses and each classification has been created for some particular purpose. In general, the purpose is practical: to help present and future (potential) patients. My aim here is not to describe the classifications, but rather to give a simple typology of diagnoses that may illustrate the large variety of them.[9,10]

A *symptom diagnosis* is the most primitive form of diagnosis. It consists of a description of a single symptom or finding. Eczema, migraine and constipation are examples of symptom diagnoses. In many instances a symptom diagnosis is simply a professional description of something that the patient already knows. Although primitive, a symptom diagnosis can be very helpful for the patient. The diagnosis of eczema, for example, gives a hint of potential treatments and the confident diagnosis of migraine excludes some more serious conditions.

Often diagnoses are defined *anatomically*. Fractures and other injuries are defined by their anatomic site but anatomical localisation is, of course, present in many kinds of diagnoses, like otitis media (middle ear infection) or oesophageal cancer.

Causal definition of a diagnosis offers a rational basis for treatment in principle and often in practice, as, for example, in the case of pneumococcal pneumonia. The concept of causality is complex and in medicine it is rarely possible to find a necessary and sufficient cause of a condition. It is not always clear which part of the causal chain is 'medical'. The proximal cause of a case of diarrhoea is often a microbe but more distal causes can be lack of clean water, poverty and an unstable political system based on former colonial exploitation. In fact, a better term to describe the phenomena would be a *web* of causation,[11] since a 'chain' may give too simplified a picture of the issue.

Medical diagnoses sometimes constitute *syndromes*. A syndrome refers to a combination of symptoms and signs. Often it is a preliminary stage in diagnosis while awaiting a more fundamental explanation. AIDS is good example of this process: it was first described as a combination of unusual findings and later on a causal agent, human immunodeficiency virus, was identified.

In many cases, syndromes are defined operationally and the patient is said to have a particular syndrome if he or she meets an agreed number of criteria for that syndrome. The criteria are often discussed in international meetings and they change when or if research progresses. This demonstrates the nature of many diagnoses: the diagnosis you have now may be different after the next meeting of the International Association of Your Diagnosis.

Sometimes syndromes are defined in a way that looks peculiar. An example is Sudden Infant Death Syndrome (SIDS):

the sudden death of an infant under one year of age which remains unexplained after a thorough case investigation, including performance of a complete autopsy, examination of the death scene, and review of the clinical history.[12]

Characteristic of medicine as an imperfect and developing practice is that in spite of the lack of knowledge about SIDS there are simple and powerful tools for preventing it. Strong evidence suggests that discouraging prone sleeping and exposure to tobacco smoke reduce the risk for SIDS greatly.[13]

SIDS represents a class of diagnoses that is common in medicine, namely *diagnoses of exclusion*. This refers to medical conditions that are described by elimination of other reasonable possibilities. Another example of such a diagnosis is *irritable bowel syndrome*, the diagnosis of Jake in one of the opening short stories of this volume.

UNIVERSALS AND NATURAL KINDS

I attended some courses in philosophy 30 years ago, just before entering medical school. As often happens with philosophy, I was hooked and have continued with philosophy ever since.

In the beginning, it was all just very interesting and fascinating, but I did not see direct connections between most of the big philosophical issues and my real life. Once I even had a conversation on this with my philosophy teacher, Professor Raili Kauppi. I remember her saying that she comes across philosophical questions frequently in her daily life.

I was taught that one of the classical problems of philosophy was the problem of *universals*. It took me over two decades to realise that this problem was alive and present in my daily life in medicine.

The Oxford Companion to Philosophy characterises the issue:

> Universals are the supposed referents of general terms like 'red', 'table' and 'tree', understood as entities distinct from any of the particular things described by those terms. But why should we suppose that such entities exist, and what must be their nature if they do?[14]

When I attended the course on the history of philosophy, this was discussed in the context of medieval philosophy, but the controversy is seen already between Plato and Aristotle. The opposite sides of the medieval discussion were *nominalists* and *realists*. The former thought that universal concepts (like cats, oranges, universities and diagnoses) did not have a meaningful existence *as such*, they were only group names for singular entities (your cat, my orange, University of Helsinki and her pneumonia). The latter thought that universal concepts exist independently from the singular entities they denote.

What does the problem of universals have to do with medicine in general and diagnoses in particular? Let me take two examples, both from my own experience.

Some years ago I came across a neighbour, an elderly lady, whom I had not seen for a while. I knew that she had had health problems and she wanted to tell her good news. The doctors had finally found out what was wrong with her, she had *fibromyalgia*.

She seemed to be very relieved about the diagnosis. The diagnosis meant that her condition was chronic but the general prognosis was good. I shared her happiness but did not share with her my scepticism about the existence of a specific disease entity called fibromyalgia.

My second example is a 14-year-old boy who came recently to a consultation with his mother, who wanted to have my opinion on her son's tantrums. After taking a careful history, my conclusion was that his problems were not medical but what he needed was some psychological support to control his behaviour in frustrating situations. His mother told me then that they had already seen a psychologist who had examined him and concluded that he had some of the characteristics of *Asperger's syndrome*.

There are internationally accepted definitions for both fibromyalgia and Asperger's syndrome, although these definitions have a tendency to be reformulated. It is questionable, however, whether they are terms that describe *natural kinds*. The question of natural kinds is another classical philosophical problem which is hard to define exactly and to which there are no final solutions. For the purposes of this paper it may be sufficient to say that:

> Natural kind terms constitute a class of general terms and include both mass terms, like 'gold' and 'water' and certain sortal terms like 'tiger' and 'apple'. Loosely, they may be said to denote types of naturally occurring stuffs and things.[15]

The same book defines *sortal* as:

> a type of term, usually a noun, e.g. 'cat' or 'person' that supplies a single principle of individuating and counting the instances it applies to.[16]

In the history of medical classification there are some famous figures who thought that diseases are natural kinds. Carl von Linne, for example, classified diseases in the same way he had successfully classified plants.

'Gold', 'water', 'tiger' and 'apple' are terms that refer to 'naturally occurring stuffs and things', but 'fibromyalgia' or 'Asperger's syndrome' hardly do so. An essential feature of the diagnosis of fibromyalgia is that it is a diagnosis of *exclusion*, i.e. it should only be made when no other medical disease can explain the symptoms.

The DSM-IV diagnostic criteria of Asperger's syndrome include, for example (italics mine),

> A. *Qualitative* impairment in social interaction, as manifested by at least two of the following:
>
> *Marked impairment* in the use of multiple nonverbal behaviours such as eye-to-eye gaze, facial expression, body postures, and gestures to regulate social interaction
>
> . . .
>
> C. The disturbance causes *clinically significant impairment* in social, occupational, or other important areas of functioning.
>
> . . .
>
> F. Criteria are not met for another specific Pervasive Developmental Disorder, or Schizophrenia.

The terms in italics demonstrate the difference between the definitions of some diagnoses and the definitions in, e.g., botany. The criterion F is again one of exclusion.

Another argument against the assumption that diagnoses were natural kinds comes from the fact that many diagnoses are defined by setting an arbitrary point on a continuum. In fact, all diagnoses that are based on continuous values of some biological variable are of this type. Three obvious examples are high blood pressure, high cholesterol and diabetes.

Even a cursory look at recent medical literature shows that indications for the treatment of all these three conditions both have changed with time and show considerable geographical variation. Since there is no obvious cut-off point that would define natural classes, the diagnosis in such cases is always an administrative decision.[17]

VALUES AND DIAGNOSES

To obtain a medical diagnosis usually means that someone has something that he or she would rather *not* have. The concept of diagnosis is thus *value-laden*. In fact, the very existence of medicine depends on an evaluation: without disease or illness there would be no medicine. Patients or at least potential patients are a precondition for medicine and medical science.

Arthur Kleinman writes about psychiatric diagnoses: 'Psychiatric diagnoses are not things, though they give name and scope to processes . . . [They] derive from categories . . . [that] are outcomes of historical development, cultural influence and political negotiation.'[18] To me it is obvious that so-called somatic diagnoses are no different. Some diagnoses are more highly evaluative than others but even the least evaluative ones are based on some prior evaluation.[19]

There are many ways to classify values and several philosophers have presented their own value typologies. My aim here is not to give an exhaustive review but just a few examples of *instrumental, epistemic, aesthetic, ethical* and *economical* values playing a role in defining and characterising diagnoses. These values are often hidden and the categories overlap but uncovering the values may reveal some important issues that are relevant even in the care of a particular patient.

Instrumental values

Instrumental values serve as means to some ends. For example, the diagnosis of *intellectual disability* as such may not be very helpful for the person in question, since it does not tell much about that person nor does it entail any specific treatment options. However, society needs information, e.g. about the prevalence of intellectual disability, to be able to plan the need for special education services. The purpose of the first test of intelligence was to identify children who were unlikely to benefit from the public education system in France.[20]

Epistemic values

Epistemic values are part of the realm of *scientific* values and concern, e.g., the certainty of judgements. An example of epistemic values playing a role in diagnostics is the diagnosis of pneumonia, which is conventionally based on chest radiography (CR). CR is often not available in outpatient clinics in the developing countries and the World Health Organization (WHO) has proposed the use of respiratory rate and chest indrawing to decide whether children presenting to outpatient clinics with cough or difficult breathing have 'clinical pneumonia'.[21] Studies have shown that CR does not necessarily add useful information to the clinical diagnosis of pneumonia.[22,23]

To make things more complicated, CR is not a good test. In one study, for example, of 26 adult pneumonia cases that were diagnosed as pneumonia using high resolution computed tomography (HRCT), only 18 were identified when using CR.[24] In another study, of six cases of pneumonia in children identified at necropsy, only three were identified by a radiologist using CR.[25] Also, the interpretation of CR to conclude that a patient has pneumonia is quite subjective.

There are thus no obvious 'objective' criteria for the diagnosis of pneumonia. Which criteria are used depend on the facilities available and the aims of the diagnosis (clinical or post-mortem diagnosis).

Aesthetic values

Many diagnoses contain overt or covert aesthetic evaluations. Being short, tall, overweight, underweight, having small or large parts in your body may all lead to medical evaluation, diagnosis and treatment. My example is tallness of young girls.

With the exception of some rare medical conditions (like pituitary adenoma), these girls are healthy. However, this has not always been obvious even to the researchers working in this area. For example, Weiman et al.[26] mentioned that, in their study population, 'none of these girls suffered from any other disease', and Peters et al.[27] wrote about 'otherwise healthy adolescent girls'.

The first scientific report of treating healthy tall girls with hormones to reduce adult height was published in 1956.[28] The treatment was considered justified because extreme tallness was 'likely to raise social and economic problems'. Since then, numerous scientific reports have been published and tens of thousands of girls treated. Obviously the enthusiasm to start treatment has varied greatly between countries, regions and individual physicians. During the past two decades societies (and parents!) have, however, become more tolerant with respect to tallness, shortness and other extremes of normal variation and a decreasing demand for this treatment has been noted by paediatric endocrinologists.

The harmfulness of tall stature in adulthood has usually been taken for granted in the medical literature. No evidence, however, has been presented to support this view. Very often the experiences of a tall mother have been the main reason treatment is sought for a tall girl.

As in the case of growth hormone for constitutionally short children or surgery for children with big ears, pharmacological treatment to prevent psycho-social harm among healthy tall girls is, in a way, treating the victims of the attitudes of families and society. This observation does not help the girls, however. Although society may have become more tolerant, pharmacological intervention may sometimes be appropriate. In the words of a paediatric endocrinologist: 'Sometimes I feel that any treatment is better than daily discussions at home about the harmfulness of tall stature.'[29]

Ethical values

Medicine is fundamentally a moral pursuit, and moral judgements can hardly be avoided in any medical activity, be it diagnostic, therapeutic or research. As an example of ethical values in the diagnostic process, consider the following example from my own clinical practice.

A Finnish couple adopted three-year-old Dimitri (not his real name) from abroad. All they know about the boy's past is that his single mother had brought him to an orphanage two years earlier. Dimitri adapted well to his new life, learned the language quickly and seemed to have a happy life. The reason he was brought to my office was a trivial infection.

When I saw Dimitri, I immediately recognised his face as a textbook example of a child with foetal alcohol syndrome (FAS). Of course, more is needed for an FAS diagnosis than a face. The other three criteria are growth retardation, prenatal alcohol exposure and brain damage. I had no growth data, nobody knew about his prenatal history and the short visit gave no hints about possible brain damage.

However, I had a moral dilemma: should I mention to his mother (about) my suspicion about FAS? Would an early diagnosis do more good than harm to Dimitri and his parents?

My decision was not to tell and the reasons were the following. During that short visit it became obvious that Dimitri was leading a normal toddler's life and did not need any medical intervention other than reassurance about the good prognosis of his minor infection. There was no major brain damage and any possible minor damage would not need attention until two years later when he would enter pre-school. At that age every child will be evaluated by a psychologist and a physician. If Dimitri had FAS, he would not have been helped by the diagnosis at the time I saw him.

Economic values

Economic values deal with the worth of things within a system of exchange in a society.[30] They are closely related to political and ethical values. My example is from prenatal diagnosis.

A common cut-off point used in the serum screening for Down's syndrome during pregnancy has been a risk of 1 in 250. A calculated risk lower than 1 in 250 is considered low. Women whose risk is higher than 1 in 250 are offered definitive prenatal diagnosis.

Economic cost-benefit analyses performed in the 1970s were an important factor in defining this particular cut-off point for screening. Maternal age was originally the only criterion used, and it was concluded that offering amnio-centesis to women 35 years and older would be cost-effective. Later, when serum screening was developed, the cut-off point of 1 in 250 was chosen because it roughly represents the risk of a 35-year-old woman. Nowadays it is less common and considered politically incorrect to refer to economic values when screening for Down's syndrome is discussed. It is worth remembering, however, that earlier, one of the main justifications for the cut-off point still in use today was cost-related.

DOES IT MATTER?

Diagnoses come and go. Occasionally, new diseases like AIDS and SARS emerge but it is more common that the labels change, not the phenomena people experience. Sick people are given different diagnoses at different times and in different places, depending on the status of science, the prevailing models of explanation and even fashion. For example, today's people are not labelled as hysterics or neurasthenics, instead they may have, for example, panic disorder, chronic fatigue syndrome (CFS) or fibromyalgia. Contemporary diagnoses reveal the things researchers are interested in today, what methods they use and what is their world view.

One diagnosis may carry different meanings to different people and receiving a diagnosis may, in fact, affect the prognosis. There is evidence that diagnosed CFS patients have a worse prognosis than fatigue syndrome patients without such a label.[31] A pessimistic illness perception after the diagnosis can become a self-fulfilling prophecy in some patients.

It is therefore legitimate to ask the question about the pros and cons of labelling patients with diagnoses like CFS. After a careful deliberation the authors conclude that the answer may turn out to depend not on the label, but on what the label implies: 'it is acceptable to make diagnoses such as CFS, provided that this is the beginning, and not the end, of the therapeutic encounter.'[32]

A clinician is usually not so much concerned about whether a particular diagnosis exists in some deep sense of the word. For her the essential question is whether the diagnosis is somehow helpful for the patient.

The meaning of diagnoses is not only an academic question. For the patient, the end of uncertainty often means that *something* can be said about the prognosis. A diagnosis of exclusion (like Jake's irritable bowel syndrome) means that the patient does *not* have certain other, often serious diagnoses like cancer.

In some cases a diagnosis may mean devastating news and many patients would probably prefer uncertainty to diagnosis. For example, a diagnosis of a motor neurone disease like amyotrophic lateral sclerosis (ALS) is such. If the diagnostic alternatives are 'arm weakness of unknown origin' and ALS, the patient may prefer the former one, presuming she knows something about ALS.

In many cases, however, the patient feels relieved when her symptoms finally get a name. This happened with my neighbour whom I described above – whatever the degree of agreement about the nature and existence of fibromyalgia within the scientific community. For her the diagnosis did matter.

REFERENCES

1 Morens DM, Katz AR. The 'fourth disease' of childhood: reevaluation of a nonexistent disease. *Am J Epidemiol.* 1991; **134**: 628–40.
2 Weisse M. The fourth disease, 1900–2000. *Lancet.* 2001; **357**: 299–301.
3 Payer L. *Medicine & Culture. Notions of health and sickness in Britain, the US, France and West Germany.* London: Victor Gollancz; 1990.
4 Clare A. National variations in medical practice. *BMJ.* 1989; **298**: 1334.
5 Engelhardt HT. *The Foundations of Bioethics.* New York/Oxford: Oxford University Press; 1986.
6 Ebrahim S. The medicalisation of old age. *BMJ.* 2002; **324**: 861–3.
7 Conrad P. The shifting engines of medicalization. *J Health Soc Behav.* 2005; **46**: 3–14.
8 Rose N. Beyond medicalisation. *Lancet.* 2007; **369**: 700–2.

9 Stempsey WE. *Disease and Diagnosis. Value-Dependent Realism.* Dordrecht: Kluwer; 2000.

10 Wulff HR. *Rational Diagnosis and Treatment.* Oxford: Blackwell; 1976.

11 Krieger N. Epidemiology and the web of causation: has anyone seen the spider? *Soc Sci Med.* 1994; **39**: 887–903.

12 www.sids.org/ndefinition.htm

13 Mitchell E. Commentary: Cot death – the story so far. *BMJ.* 1999; **319**: 1461–2.

14 Honderich T, editor. *The Oxford Companion to Philosophy.* Oxford/New York: Oxford University Press; 1995.

15 Ibid.

16 Ibid.

17 Laakso M, Groop L. Yksi, kaksi vai monta diabetesta? (*One, two or many forms of diabetes?*, in Finnish). *Duodecim.* 2007; **123**: 1427–9.

18 Cited in Bartholomew RE. *Exotic Deviance. Medicalizing Cultural Idioms from Strangeness to Illness.* Boulder, CO: University Press of Colorado; 2000.

19 Cutter MAG. *Reframing Disease Contextually.* Dordrecht: Kluwer; 2003.

20 Louhiala P. *Preventing Intellectual Disability. Ethical and Clinical Issues.* Cambridge: Cambridge University Press; 2004.

21 Pio A. Standard case management of pneumonia in children in developing countries: the cornerstone of the acute respiratory infection programme. *Bulletin of the WHO.* 2003; **81**: 298–300.

22 Swingler GH, Zwarenstein M. Chest radiograph in acute respiratory infections in children. *Cochrane Database Syst Rev.* 2005; **3**: CD001268.

23 Dirlewanger M, Krahenbuhl JD, Fanconi S *et al.* Community-acquired pneumonia in children aged 2 months to 5 years: application of the WHO guidelines in a developed country setting (Switzerland). *European Journal of Pediatrics.* 2002; **161**: 460–1.

24 Syrjälä H, Broas M, Suramo I *et al.* High resolution computed tomography for the diagnosis of community-acquired pneumonia. *Clinical Infectious Diseases.* 1998; **27**: 358–63.

25 Doherty JF, Dijkhuizen MA, Wieringa FT *et al.* WHO guidelines on detecting pneumonia in children [letter]. *Lancet.* 1991; **338**: 1454.

26 Weiman E, Bergmann S, Böhles HJ. Oestrogen treatment of constitutional tall stature: a risk-benefit ratio. *Arch Dis Child.* 1998; **78**: 148–51.

27 Peters M, ten Cate H, Sturk A. Acquired Protein S deficiency might be associated with a prethrombotic state during estrogen treatment for tall stature. *Thrombosis and Haemostasis.* 1992; **68**: 371–2.

28 Goldzieher MA. Treatment of excessive growth in the adolescent female. *J Clin Endocrin.* 1956; **16**: 249–52.

29 Louhiala P. How tall is too tall? On the ethics of oestrogen treatment of tall girls. *J Med Ethics.* 2007; **33**: 48–50.

30 Stempsey, op. cit.

31 Huibers MJH, Wessely S. The act of diagnosis: pros and cons of labelling chronic fatigue syndrome. *Psychological Medicine.* 2006; **36**: 895–900.

32 Huibers and Wessely, op. cit.

CHAPTER 7

Intimacy and distance in the clinical examination

MARTYN EVANS AND JANE MACNAUGHTON

AN INTRODUCTION, BY WAY OF FICTION

Since life so often imitates art, let us begin with art – not least, because of its ability to mislead us at first.

> Toward the end of winter, in the house of the Shcherbatskys, a consultation was being held, which was to determine the state of Kitty's health, and what was to be done to restore her failing strength. She had been ill, and, as spring came on, she grew worse. The family doctor gave her cod-liver oil, then iron, then lunar caustic; but since neither the first, nor the second, nor the third availed, and since his advice was to go abroad before the beginning of the spring, a celebrated doctor was called in. The celebrated doctor, not yet old and a very handsome man, demanded an examination of the patient. He maintained, with special satisfaction, it seemed, that maidenly modesty is merely a relic of barbarism, and that nothing could be more natural than for a man who was not yet old to handle a young girl in the nude. He deemed this natural, because he did it every day, and neither felt nor thought, as it seemed to him, anything evil as he did it and, consequently, he considered girlish modesty not merely as a relic of barbarism, but, as well, an insult to himself.

It was necessary to submit, for, although all the doctors studied in the same school, all using the same textbooks, and all learned in the same science, and though some people said this celebrated doctor was but a poor doctor, in the Princess's household and circle it was for some reason held that this celebrated doctor alone had some peculiar knowledge, and that he alone could save Kitty. After thorough examination and tapping of the patient, distraught and dazed with shame, the celebrated doctor, having painstakingly washed his hands, was standing in the drawing room talking to the Prince. The Prince frowned and coughed as he listened to the doctor. As a man who had seen something of life, and neither a fool nor an invalid, he had no faith in medicine, and at soul was wrought up with all this comedy, especially as he was probably the only one who fully understood the cause of Kitty's illness. 'You're barking up the wrong tree,' he mentally applied this phrase from the hunter's vocabulary to the celebrated doctor, as he listened to the latter's patter about the symptoms of his daughter's complaint. The doctor, for his part, found difficulty in restraining the expression of his contempt for this old grandee, as well as in condescending to the low level of his comprehension. He perceived that it was useless to talk to the old man, and that the head of this house was the mother – and she it was before whom he intended to scatter his pearls. It was at this point that the Princess entered the drawing room with the family doctor. The Prince retreated, doing his best not to betray how ridiculous he regarded the whole comedy. The Princess was distraught, and did not know what to do. She felt herself at fault before Kitty.

'Well, doctor, decide our fate,' said the Princess. 'Tell me everything.' – 'Is there any hope?' was what she had wanted to say, but her lips quivered, and she could not utter this question. 'Well, doctor?'

'Immediately, Princess – I will discuss the matter with my colleague, and then have the honour of laying my opinion before you.'

'Then we had better leave you?'

'As you please.'

The Princess, with a sigh, stepped outside.[1]

Perhaps it is characteristic of the highest levels of literary creation that a text bears several plausible interpretations; perhaps it is characteristic of enthusiastic readers that our initial understanding may be simplistic, to be discarded in favour of later and subtler readings. At first sight, Tolstoy seems to have a simple target – the cynical violation of a young woman's sexual modesty by an exploitative and powerful professional; certainly this is the immediate focus of

Kitty's shame and anger. However things may be by no means so simple.

To begin with, it's not clear that the celebrated specialist consciously intends either violation or his own gratification, at least not of any sexual nature. Tolstoy is naturally ambiguous about this. What the specialist's unconscious motive is may give the lie to his conscious self-directed assurances, and we are told he appears to reserve 'special satisfaction' for these particular assurances ('satisfaction' here has available to it at least the bawdy ambiguity of a Restoration comedy if not yet quite the strictures of Freud). But we do not need to judge the matter, for more is at stake than the sexual. The specialist enjoys power, whatever else he enjoys: the power among other things to make what would be outrageous for others natural and inevitable for himself. This is a form of gratification that he has conveniently arranged for himself on a daily basis. But it expresses itself in other ways – his contempt for his paying customers and their ignorance, those before whom he 'scatters his pearls'. Tolstoy's own outrage seems ultimately more directed at this than at the scandalising of a girl's modesty which, although clearly instrumental to the specialist's self-indulgence, need not itself constitute the ulterior motive that, in turn, scandalises Tolstoy – or us.

For we *are* scandalised – and rightly. But what is at stake is not sexual exploitation so much as the reckless disregard of sexual respect: not so much the violation of sexual intimacy as the violation of intimacy *per se*. The intimacy whose violation underlies Kitty's understandable distress and sense of shame is the intimacy of presumption. Neither her physical nakedness nor her helpless cooperation (Tolstoy tells us she was obliged 'to submit') should have been the doctor's to command, yet command it he did, and worse still with a faint air of having himself been injured by the whiff of outdated squeamishness that dares to defy his professional access to Kitty's body, his supposed medical *droit de seigneur*.

And from art, let us turn to life.

THE PHYSICAL EXAMINATION

This chapter considers the physical examination in clinical medicine, and in particular the first such examination in a newly-emerging illness, or in a new episode of a prior illness. We aim to consider what is required in terms of the relationship between doctor and patient for an examination to take place appropriately, and what being 'examined' – in some sense like an object – means for the patient's body and its ordinary standing within the world. In exploring this we will consider notions of intimacy and distance and what these mean in the professional-patient relationship. But first we must consider what is meant by the medical examination, be it in a physical or a psychiatric context.

Although a physical examination is normally preceded by dialogue, and normally involves close visual attention – both capable of giving rise to considerations of intimate matters – the fact remains that when we think about the physical examination in medicine we immediately think about touch. More specifically we think about the doctor touching the patient in a manner that would be uncomfortable (psychologically as well as, perhaps, physically) if done by anyone else outside the context of a relationship that is already, and for other reasons, physically intimate. Such relationships may be those between lovers, or between parents and children; in every case the ages of the parties are important in relation to matters of both consent and stage of physical development. Some forms of touching might be thought by many to be entirely unacceptable outside a medical context.

Consider one of our fictional patients, Jake, who experiences profound embarrassment when he has to undergo a rectal examination by his female doctor. We do not hear much about what the doctor felt but assume a professional neutrality about the event – and we hear her acknowledge his discomfort by apologising for having to put him through this indignity. However, before the doctor puts a hand on the patient other forms of examination are going on. We have already discussed verbal examination: the taking of a case history and the attempt to establish a shared meaning and understanding about what the problem is. Just as in any exchange or meeting between two human beings, so too the conversation that produces the case history also involves the establishing of a relationship, if doctor and patient have not met before, or the extending of it, if they have met and engaged previously. Little things get noticed by both parties that lead to judgements about what kind of person each might be. In Rachel's story we get some evidence of this. Rachel has noticed some things about the doctor: she 'always looked tired', her hair was 'scruffed up in a clip', 'she waved her hands a lot'. These characteristics help Rachel to form a view about the doctor and she seems at ease with her and trusts her. Doctors will notice similar mundane things about patients before turning on the more professional, conscious gaze that is the first prerequisite of the physical examination.

From the doctor's perspective, medical students are always taught that examination starts the moment the patient enters the room. Students are encouraged to observe the patient's demeanour, their gait, other movements and their ability to make eye contact – or otherwise. As far as the patient is concerned, however, the examination starts when they are invited to present part of their body to be looked at, touched, manipulated and listened to by the doctor. At this point their familiar, everyday body begins a subtle change in status, becoming what has been called the 'medical body', an object sub-mitted to the professional medical gaze.[2] We shall consider this a little further, below, but for now it is enough to notice the distinction from the body of daily experience that this crucial abstraction involves.

The abstraction is crucial because it would otherwise seem extraordinary that this amount of intimate handling of one person's flesh by another can take place when in some circumstances the two people have only just met, as seems the case in Jake's story. It is unthinkable in the circumstances of ordinary human relationships where friendship and even love are normally prereq-uisites for such intimate contact. The irony within the patient-professional relationship is that such intimate physical contact is possible in circumstances where friendship and love does not exist – or indeed that, in the particularly 'clinical' form, it may be possible especially, even if not only, where they do not exist.

There is more to this than touch alone, of course. The medical examina-tion can be physically intimate through what is seen as well as through what is touched, and it can be psychologically intimate through what is said and heard. More than one mode of intimacy can be at stake simultaneously; and certainly a consultation that goes awry can be both physically and psychologi-cally humiliating. Bertolt Brecht, writing of a more systematically callous age, condemns the dual shame of physical and circumstantial suffering endured by patients who are also paupers, undergoing a clinical examination involving the doctor's eyes and ears with neither insight nor imagination:

> When we visit you
> Our clothes are ripped and torn
> And you listen all over our naked body.
> As to the cause of our illness
> A glance at our rags would be more
> Revealing. One and the same cause wears out
> Our bodies and our clothes.[3]

Pride taken in appearance is the reverse of shame at poverty disclosed; the worker-patients described by Brecht have their dignity ripped from them along with their clothes, and twice over at that. Most of us are fortunate to live in gentler times, economically speaking, but our vulnerabilities take other forms, and intimacy sometimes consists in disclosing our softer parts in psychological as well as – or instead of – physical terms.

For example, consider a clinical encounter which did not involve physical examination. This encounter forms the central part of a novel by Salley Vickers called *The Other Side of You*.[4] In the first part of the novel a psychiatrist, David McBride, attempts in various ways to get his suicidal patient to explain how it was that she reached the point of very nearly succeeding in taking her own life. He describes how his examination of his patients begins in their first session:

> I would tend to spend the first session with any new patient asking pretty mundane questions, hoping I was absorbing the myriad clues which human beings give off even in the simplest transactions: the set of the head, or the jaw, or the shoulders, the arms folded or relaxed, the play of the hands, the flicker of the eyelids, the pallor of the skins, the way the feet make contact with the ground, the pitch of the voice – crucial, for me, I find – the choice of vocabulary, the pace and cadence of the words, how the eyes would meet yours or look away. (p. 11)

He notices such subtle aspects of his patient in such a way that he is able to make certain judgements about her character and her likely responses to him. But it takes time and a number of fruitless consultations before he takes a risk, and introduces a note to their conversation that seems to overstep the professional relationship into a more intimate friendship relationship. He apologises for cancelling the previous consultation and she responds:

> 'It doesn't matter.'
> 'If you say not.'
> 'It's not important.' This time I held my peace. 'I don't make the mistake of assuming I matter to you!' She broke out suddenly again, with more than a hint of sharpness. (p. 74)

Here, the doctor seems to have overstepped the mark and allowed a different relationship to develop between himself and his patient, one that has raised in this patient the expectation of mutual regard. But by allowing this he also opens the floodgates to her story and ultimately to her cure. As she tells her story we observe their relationship deepen and become even more intimate. The only barrier that remains between them is a physical one and as readers we feel that if they were to touch physically, then the doctor-patient relationship – and Elizabeth's cure – would become impossible.

ASPECTS OF INTIMACY IN THE CLINICAL RELATIONSHIP

On the face of it, we think of intimacy as a good thing, valuable, desirable, a mark of attainment in a relationship of friendship or love; but it appears in other contexts as well and some of these may be highly aversive. Intimacy is capable of being exploited, as when friends fall out and become spiteful or vengeful. Or it is capable of being recruited into something that is already damaging and dangerous. An oppressive or exploitative or manipulative relationship (perhaps in the context of employment) becomes intensified by the imposition of intimacy upon the unwilling party. Or intimacy can start out as damaging – the relationship between the torturer and his victim is nothing if not intimate, typically in a bodily sense, sometimes in a psychological sense as well.

Intimacy can be carefully prepared and cultivated over time, or it can be casual. It has been suggested that women, more so than men, will readily share intimate *information* with comparative strangers (other women) on first meeting.[5] And both men and women are familiar with the phenomenon of significant and relatively intimate conversations with people whom one is unlikely ever to meet again – the phenomenon of 'aeroplane friends'.

Intimacy in the sense of emotional closeness (whether in the context either of sexual or of platonic relations) is also mutual, reciprocal. We cannot be emotionally intimate with another if they are not also emotionally intimate with us; one-sided attempts at intimacy can result in self-deception, of course, on the part of the would-be intimate, but the genuine article requires a corresponding will and engagement from both parties.

Considering these aspects of intimacy in the clinical relationship, we may perhaps begin by excluding sexual relations simply because of their obvious and indeed banal impermissibility in this context. Let us instead consider simply *closeness*. Closeness itself has many relevant senses for the clinician. They include closeness of observation (as in, significantly, what we often call *intimate* knowledge of a subject, personal or impersonal); the strict keeping of confidences (something that is self-evidently needed between clinician and patient); rapport (the foundation, perhaps, of a sense of common purpose); the acceptance of a degree of familiarity (but within limits – not casual personal familiarity so much as a shared understanding and knowledge).

There is one other, intriguing, aspect of this: friendliness and friendship are both manifestations of closeness, but it's important that these are not the same thing, and whilst friendliness in the sense of cordiality seems an important part of any well-tempered civil transaction, friend*ship* does not seem either necessary or desirable. Thurstan Brewin, a clinician who spent his career caring for the terminally ill, described his understanding of 'professional friendliness':

> Professional friendship is not quite the same as ordinary friendship, but much that applies still holds true. A friend is warm and welcoming at each meeting. A friend pays small compliments . . . A friend is just as ready to talk seriously (if that is what the patient wants) as to joke or gossip. A really supportive friend does not go over the top emotionally, but is always concerned; doesn't stay too long; knows when to be silent; doesn't ask too many questions. A doctor should follow suit.[6]

Brewin characterises the supportive relationship of doctor to patient in this way in order to point out that no special training is required. He emphasises that this friendliness should derive from the authentic interest of the clinician and not from the rules of communication skills courses. This extract characterises the manner of the doctor's approach: it is *like* friendship; the doctor acts in the way a friend would act, but is not a friend in the way the patient's other friends might be. It would be inappropriate for the doctor, for example, to join the patient for a pint in the pub, or to invite her round for dinner or out to the cinema, even if those actions might help relieve the patient's symptoms for a while or soothe her fear of illness. The doctor may need to reach underneath his professional persona to find an appropriately authentic friendly approach, but it is still different from the kind of closeness implied by true friendship. It is friendship at a distance.

Clinical intimacy then, we might say (echoing Wittgenstein's notion of the dispassionate conduct of philosophical enquiry as residing in a 'cool place')[7] needs to be an intimacy of a peculiarly 'cool' form. So we will suggest the expression 'cool intimacy' as a way of capturing the apparently inconsistent demands of intimacy in the clinical context, combining the unusually close physical or perceptual proximity of doctor and patient with the necessary psychological detachment and 'safe' distance between them in emotional terms.

This is an essentially bloodless form of intimacy, and it's normally necessary that it be so. As such, 'cool intimacy' can be confined to (and hence can serve) a mutually agreed, and professionally-proper, purpose. It is temporarily disturbing but is intended to be ultimately safe, and is entered into on that expectation.

Of course this is a general statement, and there can be exceptions to it. Comfort and care are always at least implicitly a part of medicine. So an interesting question arises as to whether *professional* care is always 'cool' in the sense that we've defined it. Consider for instance those clinical contexts where coolness did not help – in the case of children, in connection with certain kinds of psychological disorders, or in rehabilitation and other contexts where the warmth of personal encouragement could be therapeutically important. Nonetheless the coolness of clinical intimacy seems to be a useful place to start in considering the typical context of physical examinations of adult patients. The coolness forms part of an answer to the perennial question of what kinds of affective components are involved in professional care – whether 'caring for' involves 'caring about' in an emotional sense, when this is what one does professionally. It also addresses the potency of physical contact, touch, which must be 'cool' in the sense of being dispassionate and detached and, so far as possible, objective for the purposes of rational diagnosis – even whilst acknowledging that touch in *healing* needs also to be experienced by the patient as 'warm' in the existential sense, as a manifestation of contact between people whose goodwill and kindly purposes are embodied within that contact.

Of course, the range of expressions of kindly purposes is wide – wider than professional ethics would ordinarily allow. In Robertson Davies's *The Cunning Man*, Dr Jonathan Hullah and his formidable assistant deal with suspected hypochondria through the jaunty withering of the modesty of Miss Fothergill, a middle-aged spinster, recounted unsympathetically by one of Hullah's female friends:

> Before she even saw the great man she had quite a session with the dragon, Nurse Christofferson. All the usual details recorded on paper, and whisked into the examination-room and ordered to strip, and not just to her undies, but ballock-naked which she made sound utterly horrible; she has an awful lot of shame for a rather small woman. Then up on that platform I told you about, and Christofferson disappeared under the black cloth of a big camera like an old-fashioned portrait camera, and turns on several cruel and searching lights

and takes her picture in a wide variety of unbecoming poses. 'I trust that these pictures are confidential,' sez La Fothergill. 'Yes,' sez Christofferson with more humour than I would have expected, 'any views you want for sale or distribution must be taken elsewhere.'[8]

For a really savage account of the use of the clinical examination as a curiously scrupled form of humiliation – albeit in what seems to be a medically-justified cause – see the increasingly ruthless remainder of the passage just quoted. All of which reminds us that the notion of intimacy raises, throughout, questions of where the boundaries of professional care and engagement lie. These boundaries must recognise the necessary closeness of perceptual and physical contact, and of a sufficient distance in psychological engagement – a distance allowing separateness or distinctness of will and purpose. The wills and purposes of the patient and clinician must sufficiently align, without this being mistaken for the subjugation of one party by the other. Clinical cool intimacy involves a form of concession on both parties, compared with ordinary interpersonal engagement. The patient loans his body for the purposes of close examination, and in return the physician temporarily surrenders a part of her ordinary repertoire of reactions and responses, retaining only those appropriate to examination and diagnosis. How these concessions can be made is something we shall consider a little later on.

But meanwhile let us consider 'cool intimacy' in the examination of our four patients.

OUR FOUR PATIENTS
Rachel

First, Rachel. Aside from any twinges she might have with regard to a general physical examination – and at the age of ten this might reasonably be quite minimal – there could be a specific embarrassment connected with investigating urinary habits and the production of a urine sample. In addition there could be what we might call a form of referred embarrassment concerning the disclosure of what she had kept hidden, which includes petty thieving in her own home. Perhaps it is easier to discuss this with a clinician than with her mother. There are clearly verbal as well as other forms of intimacy, and admitting inappropriate behaviour (however understandable) requires this. It's an extension perhaps of what we could call 'moral intimacy' in any confessional context.

Cool intimacy perhaps offers little to Rachel, given her age. Warmth and understanding are more important. However, if it is indeed easier to discuss the 'confessional' aspects of her illness with the doctor than with her mother, this suggests that a certain coolness is important to moral intimacy.

Jake

Next, Jake – and for someone with two embarrassing conditions (psoriasis and irritable bowel) cool intimacy seems highly desirable. The clinician's access to Jake's body needs to contrast as strongly as possible with the access that Jake would like to be able to offer to his hoped-for girlfriend Carol but, for the time being, dare not. The whole point is that the clinician does not need to *approve* Jake's body in any usual sense – admiration, emulation, appreciation, desire, etc. If s/he approves Jake's body in a more intellectual sense it will be as a resource for clinically interesting or noteworthy features – much as the crossword addict would approve a particularly thorny problem or the collector appreciate a rare butterfly.

Of course this puzzler's or collector's interest in Jake's body is *a fortiori* a peculiar manifestation of cool intimacy. Indeed we might even say that the coolness lies in the intellectualisation of engagement as distinct from the emotional (or appetitive) forms of engagement. It is also a special kind of abstraction from Jake's lived condition. We'll come back to this, below; and meanwhile we should insist that this puzzler's or collector's interest is not a necessary feature of the 'clinical gaze'. It might, however, be a usual one.

With or without that collector's interest, the clinical gaze tends to assimilate reported descriptions along with observed signs into evidence for rational diagnosis. This is a forensic interest in the body – the body as evidence. By constituting another way in which the clinician meets Jake's body intellectually rather than emotionally, it can call upon cool intimacy.

Liz

When we're introduced to Liz the immediate context is a prospective smear test, perhaps as intimate a clinical consultation as could readily be imagined. However this is incidental to her underlying problem, epilepsy; intimacy here concerns both the clinical response to an acute episode – convulsions and fainting – and the general, considered, long-term management of the condition.

Like Jake, Liz has bodily sources of embarrassment (since a fit may involve incontinence, for instance) but it seems clear that her epilepsy is a source of a more existential embarrassment, even shame. The fits produce confusion and temporary dysphasia; living with the condition and its propensity to result in fits from time to time has over the course of the illness induced her, regularly, to lie – she is an habitual liar, 'like a trooper', in search of leading a life that others will be persuaded to perceive as normal and hence, presumably, reliable – reliable enough, for instance, to retain custody of her daughter.

Cool intimacy would help in defusing the consequences of incontinence, even the reported consequences, later on; it would appear greatly preferable to the nurse's shocked and somehow apologetic stare. The apology compounds the shock; it reinforces the fact of shock and its causes, causes that lie within Liz. The expression of shock is an emotional disclosure, however unbidden – a reluctant intimacy that Liz could do without. The apology can be both an belated attempt to restore distance, and an admission that distance was not there when it was needed.

Jen

For Jen there are in effect three clinical contexts. Two involve her GP, Dr Gaitens: he cares both for her and for Geoff, her husband, whose confusion and intellectual deterioration following a stroke require from Jen a level of patience and forbearance that Dr Gaitens recognises and appreciates. The third context, at the time we meet Jen, lies in the near future, the much-feared hospital appointment whose postal notification nearly brings her to her knees.

Gaitens knows she's afraid; he knows also how wearying she finds caring for Geoff: to convey these concerns between doctor and patient in any meaningful way is to take us beyond cool intimacy, at least in these specific regards. Genuine concern for an individual personally known to us is akin to the moral intimacy of friends; genuine concern is liable to begin in emotional warmth, even if time and circumstances force distance upon it. Gaitens has to disentangle this from his professional concern to subject Jen to the necessary clinical investigations as soon as possible, despite – even because of – her fears.

We don't yet know whether Jen's more elderly age will make her additionally sensitive about clinical examinations, or *per contra* more phlegmatic and resigned to minor indignities; after all, she has survived intact a war and its austere aftermath. So it may be that, at the hospital, her mortal fears are the most vivid features in the consultation and investigation. An experienced clinician may be able to afford a little warmth in responding to this: acknowledging and absorbing someone's fear is surely an intimate act, whatever else it is.

PROFESSIONAL DISTANCE

Medical or clinical 'professional distance' is to be distinguished from other kinds of inter-personal distance. Your personal space can be invaded by any-one, regardless of professional role. If – broadly speaking – we dislike this invasion (and it seems to be a near-universal natural instinct to dislike it) then the question is whether the professional clinician has special respon-sibilities not to do what we dislike. Presumably the answer is a qualified 'yes' – the qualification coming in the form of consent – since a great deal of what we might expect in healthcare (exposure, discomfort, injections, pills) is liable to be at least minimally disliked. So if in general a consent legitimates what follows it, a specific consent can specifically legitimate the invasion of personal space (among any other infringements of ordinary inter-personal distance). The consent must come with a price: it must be conditional, in that the professional must among other things agree to limit the ordinary range of personal dimensions of the encounter, presumably also replacing some of these dimensions with specific aspects such as intelligent, detached, purposive observation and so on.

The distance is achieved by replacing the personal with the impersonal, or depersonalised. But this can happen only up to a point: complete deper-sonalisation would be grotesque, perhaps horrific, were it possible. (As a very incomplete instance of this, imagine a clinician rendered 'faceless' by the implacable wearing of a surgical mask throughout every encounter whether hygienically necessary or not.) Short of complete depersonalisation, how much is right? Is it settled in advance by protocol, or negotiated at the time, or a mixture of both?

Recall that professional distance has always been made possible by the nature of the consultation. Once, histories were taken and diagnoses were made *by correspondence*. Correspondence can of course be highly intimate, as lovers know to their delight or to their disgrace, depending upon circum-stances; for the possibilities and limitations of such medicine-by-epistle, see the engaging review by Louis-Courvoisier and Mauron.[9] Later, technologies interposed between the patient's body and the doctor's body – recall Roy Porter's perceptive account of Laennec's patient and the introduction of the stethoscope[10] – such that the physician's physical intimacy with the patient's body was to that extent bypassed, made redundant or at least replaced by an intimacy that was now part-mechanical.

The history of the technologies of consultation is very largely the history of the forms taken by 'professional distance'.

INTIMACY AND 'THE MEDICAL BODY'

Gillett makes the point that it is a pity that medical students do not begin to learn the art of clinical examination by examining conscious patients with neurological conditions, because standardly such patients are collaboratively involved in reporting the effects of tests and interventions in real time, rather than simply observed as in many other clinical areas.[11] This reminds us that in certain contexts, including some clinical contexts, *just looking at* someone is much more threatening than looking at them whilst talking to them, collaborating with them, interacting generally. These other aspects of engaging with another person supply limits to the range of possible expectations and emotions – 'mind sets' – that might arise during the act of looking at them; they can limit the looking to forms that are appropriate. Without such limits, our normal expectations are cut adrift and we are isolated, uncertain and vulnerable.

Something like this is at stake when as patients we submit to being viewed, for a time, primarily as physical objects. This peculiarly medical form of viewing is at some level an indispensable part of the rational understanding of disease, and of the necessary detachment that makes such rationality the ground of 'correct compassion' in Kirkup's phrase.[12] Whilst as patients we know it to be necessary, this 'medical gaze' is both reassuring as it emanates from an expert understanding and at the same time *disturbing*, reminding us at some level that though our bodies constitute the presentation of the world to us, for other people we are simply one object among many others *within* their worlds. In this sense the notion of the 'medical gaze' is already quite disturbing enough, without generalising it to the forms of institutional control that Foucault had in mind when using the phrase.[13] Well short of that general form of oppression, the medical gaze can objectify in an insulting manner, as was Kitty's experience in the passage from Tolstoy with which we began. Her well-being is subordinated to the doctor's ego, her recovery to his reputation and fortune. It is a short step from there to those other demeaning, even predatory, 'objectifying' gazes as when a labourer, a model or an athlete is visually assessed by someone wanting to make use solely of their physical capabilities and characteristics, or when someone is visually surveyed for his or her sexual desirability without regard for their personhood or their dignity.

Hence the importance of talking, listening, answering and asking questions so as to guide and interpret one's gaze when it falls upon another person, and hence also Gillett's preference for teaching clinical examination in the essentially inter-personal context of neurological diagnosis.

What are the medical bodies of our four patients? They are, of course, abstractions from the four individuals – the bodies wear those individuals' names as labels. They are biological organisms, varying to some extent from the normal type (allowing for age and sex). They are the loci of disease processes. They 'belong to' the people whose names they bear in a relation almost of ownership rather than identity, of detachment (for the time being) rather than integrity. In Rachel, the child with diabetes enduring a crisis of shame and anxiety becomes the case of childhood diabetes; in Liz, the mother struggling with both epilepsy and self-esteem becomes the epileptic female. These medical bodies (and those of Jen and Jake) consist in their respective deficiencies, first and foremost.

Of course this is, in the context of understanding their problems, fair enough to begin with, although incomplete. One basis of the medical body, following Byron Good, is that it is an *abstraction from the 'life-world'*. This awkward notion, elegantly explored by Good,[14] refers to a collective (and perhaps collectively-unconscious) habit of medical rationality – the intentional isolation of the patient-as-organism from its context in daily life insofar as that context extends beyond the reach of bio-scientific description. (It is perhaps ironic that 'the life-world' in this sense should so elude the life-sciences!) Such an abstraction is the consequence of retreating, or reducing, from the lived body of the patient to 'the medical body'. At stake is the danger of loss of meaning (existential meaning, experiential reality) from whatever phenomena are presented to the doctor. After the abstraction, what is left is meant to be something that biomedicine can deal with – the impassion'd clay relieved of its passion, and now reduced just to the clay alone. But our sceptical presumption is that, even if it be intelligible (and it may not be), working with the clay alone is often insufficient, perhaps even harmful, particularly if the patient's experiential problem is left to persist, whilst the criteria of biomedicine have been satisfied and the patient to that extent dismissed. This seems to be what happens to Oliver Sacks after the surgery on his knee (*A Leg to Stand On*).[15]

The abstraction has both a medico-cultural and an epistemological form. The epistemological abstraction is needed in order to *make sense of* what is seen. Medical science deals in the ways in which patients are – or ought to be – all alike: departures from the statistical norms for structure and function are the coinage of scientific diagnosis. We will leave aside here the enormous problem of combining this with the individuality of the patient, something that tops the epistemological agenda for the medical humanities, we take it. The epistemological abstraction gains for us a measure of understanding. But obtaining it requires this other abstraction, the medico-cultural abstraction, which makes it possible to *look, touch and act with immunity* from the ordinary constraints of intimacy. It is a kind of defence against intimacy, a defence on the part of and in the interests of the doctor as much as the patient. And why should not the doctor preserve his or her own emotional balance by a sort of abstraction from psychological intimacy? Perhaps the medical body is precisely one that allows physical intimacy without its psychological counter-part – a psychologically-distancing manoeuvre, a psychologically-distancing phenomenon, that is (to borrow again from Kirkup) the true concomitant of the calm reflection needed for diagnosis.[16] An emotionally-drained clinician is not much use to man or beast.

Thus the doctor also needs – to an extent – to inhabit a kind of 'medical body' herself, whilst within the clinical context. Abstracting the patient's medi-cal body is one defence against the implications of intimacy; retreating to one's own 'medical body' may be another. The abstraction of the medical body from the patient-as-a-whole involves a manageable amount of depersonalisation – a reduction – in the direction of a machine without its 'ghost'[17] (the ghost is left with what we might call verbal reporting duties[18]). But perhaps this deperson-alisation makes sense for the clinician as well.

Clearly it could during technical procedures. Machines can make direct physical contact without tears; the clinician as manipulator of the machines (we include here the stethoscope) is the guiding intelligence, attuned to the machine and its object, part of the procedure rather than the master of cer-emonies, the driver of the bus rather than a fellow-passenger or tour host. Passengers must not speak to the driver without good reason nor distract his attention whilst the bus is in motion.

But that is to serve a technical purpose. Some measure of retreat to her *own* medical body on the part of the clinician protects her as well as the patient; it renders both into the common coin of organisms, defective or sound as the case may be – so paradoxically there is a kind of sympathetic bond on this rather primitive level. When Jake's doctor performs the digital rectal examina-tion upon him, both doctor and patient are in that moment acutely aware of the necessary *retreat* that each has made within a 'medical body' of one kind or another. In so doing, the clinician's individuality is partly obscured or sup-pressed as well as is the patient's. We may or may not think this a good thing in the clinical encounter, and we may remain puzzled regardless of whether we have ethics or epistemology in mind.

In the end, the sheer fact that our living embodiment, the locus of experience, can be approached, modified (for good or ill), or temporarily disregarded, *is* on one level puzzling to us. This is one of the most puzzling parts of the often-puzzling role that, as patients, we ask our doctors to play. We ask them to remain engaged with us in shared human understanding of our problems and our frailties, and we ask them also to disengage from us in intimate examination of us, suspending – in the interests of our dignity and their own – the usual mutual acknowledgement that would, at this level of intensity, be both shocking and threatening. As Rudebeck put it, '[this] abstraction . . . [this] coolness is then the morally qualified effort to come to grips with the factual predicament of the patient.'[19] The retreat into the medical body makes intimacy safe.

To think of what we have discussed above – the 'medical bodies' as inhabited by both doctor and patient – as static phenomena within a clinical consultation would, however, be too simplistic. At various points during a consultation, both doctor and patient will experience themselves and the transaction between them a number of different ways. Jake's ability to endure the rectal examination was possible because he was able in some sense to retreat from inhabiting the body that was being entered and defiled in this way. Once the examination was over, he returned to it, aware of his physical presence and of his cheeks burning. The doctor experiences this same kind of retreat during the act of examining. 'Just relax,' she says, professionally aware that a tense patient will contract the muscles of the anal sphincter and make the examination difficult, but, as a person with the same physiology as the patient, *physically* aware of this too. As she begins the examination, however, her awareness of her own feeling body must retreat as professional considerations take over: assessing the information from her probing finger, digging a little deeper, despite perhaps some reluctant noises and tightenings from the patient, because she knows the importance of excluding a cancerous lump. Both doctor and patient will oscillate between awareness and retreat from their own embodiment depending on what is happening at any one time in the transaction. This is a complex feat for us to undertake, but ensures that we can retreat when necessary when our embodiment becomes unbearable, and then return to face up to its implications.

A 'FAILURE OF ORDINARY DISTANCE'

Finally, intimacy and distance in the clinical consultation draw us back to the notion that illness disrupts our expectations of the ordinary. Partly these are expectations of what we can *do*, as Fulford first observed.[20] But partly they are also expectations of one can simply *be*.[21]

Such failures in our ordinary daily being appear not merely in the intrinsic symptoms of illness – pain, nausea, breathlessness, weakness – but in what we might call its *circumstantial* symptoms as well, including dependence, vulnerability or the loss of dignity, whose chief manifestation is that to a greater or lesser extent one loses the right to control or withhold intimacy. One may retain this right in law, but that is of rather theoretical interest when facing the need for an intimate examination either physical or psychological: our sense of control over our own intimacy is undermined, and in the practical circumstances of an encounter between two people this is precisely the control that matters.

In illness and in the clinical consultation, our ordinary modesty and our ordinary dignity are liable to fail, as we confront our own material and existential vulnerability in the company of the physician to whom we present it. (This may be merely temporary for the purposes of the clinical consultation, though the diagnosis may mean something more permanent.) While circumstances require it, our ordinary dignity and modesty are suspended and replaced by a kind of fiction, a constructed dignity created for the purpose. This is the nominal, almost honorific, dignity afforded within 'cool intimacy' as we have described it, and when it is all that we can cling to, cling to it we assuredly will.

REFERENCES

1 Tolstoy L. *Anna Karenina* (1876). Reprinted as *Anna Karenin*, trans. R Edmonds. Harmondsworth: Penguin; 1954.

2 Good B. *Medicine, Rationality and Experience*. Cambridge: Cambridge University Press; 1994.

3 Brecht B. [stanza from] 'A Worker's speech to a Doctor' (1936), reproduced in Bamforth I. *The Body in the Library*. London: Verso; 2003, pp. 167–8.

4 Vickers S. *The Other Side of You*. London: Harper Perennial; 2007.

5 Gallop C, personal communication.

6 Brewin T. *The Friendly Professional*. Bognor Regis: Eurocommunica Publications; 1996; pp. 74–9.

7 For example, Phillips DZ. *Philosophy's Cool Place*. Ithaca, NY: Cornell University Press; 1999.

8 Davies R. *The Cunning Man*. Harmondsworth: Penguin; 1995, pp. 274–5.

9 Louis-Courvoisier M, Mauron A. 'He found me very well; for me, I was still feeling sick.' The strange worlds of physicians and patients in the 18th and 21st centuries. *J Med Ethics: Medical Humanities*. 2002; **28**: 9–13.

10 Porter R. *Cambridge Illustrated History of Medicine*. Cambridge: Cambridge University Press; 1996; p. 174 (note to plate on p. 175).

11 Gillett G, personal communication.

12 Kirkup J. 'A Correct Compassion', from his *A Correct Compassion and Other Poems*. Oxford: Oxford University Press; 1952.

13 Foucault M. *The Birth of the Clinic: an archaeology of medical perception*, trans. A Sheridan. London: Tavistock; 1973.

14 Good B, op. cit.

15 Sacks O. *A Leg to Stand On*. London: Duckworth; 1984.

16 Kirkup J, op. cit.

17 Ryle G. *The Concept of Mind*. London: Hutchinson; 1949.

18 Evans M. Pictures of the patient: medicine, science and humanities. In: M Evans and K Sweeney. *The Human Side of Medicine*. London: Royal College of General Practitioners; 1998.

19 Rudebeck CE, personal communication.

20 Fulford KWM. *Moral Theory and Medical Practice*. Cambridge: Cambridge University Press; 1990.

21 Evans HM. Music, interrupted. In: M Evans, R Ahlzén, I Heath and J Macnaughton, editors. *Medical Humanities Companion. Volume 1 Symptom*. Oxford: Radcliffe Publishing; 2008, pp. 14–26.

CHAPTER 8

The physician's understanding of the patient's bodily meaning

CARL-EDVARD RUDEBECK

ABOUT THE CHAPTER

This chapter is about the role of bodily empathy in making a clinical diagno-sis, and for clinical communication in a broader sense. It begins with some comments on intersubjectivity in general, after which I outline some recent scientific perspectives on intersubjectivity. I trace empathy back to its origin in German hermeneutics, and then look at it from a phenomenological perspec-tive. I also discuss the contribution of imagination to the empathetic processes. In the final section, I think about empathy in the clinic with an emphasis on the bodily dimension of empathy. The chapter concludes by reading Anne MacLeod's patient stories through the lens of bodily empathy.

INTERSUBJECTIVITY

Understanding is just a milder degree of misunderstanding. This is a solipsis-tic and clearly pessimistic view on communication, based in a philosophical tradition that maintains that all you really know is that which goes on in your own mind. Nonetheless, a solipsist, George Berkeley,[1] wrote extensively about his ideas, although, of course, the deepest message of these ideas was that they had no bearing on the experiences of others. Berkeley's academic conviction was of logical character, but he lived the natural conviction that communication – ideas, experiences – between minds is possible. But, brought to the extreme, even the natural standpoint, saying that communication simply *is*, without complication, loses sight of the fact that humans communicate with varying degrees of involvement, richness and intention. Communication works, and it fails, in a fashion that is not either/or. Scepticism as questioning makes sense. It inspires an examination of the conditions of communication. In the gap of insecurity, an utterance may either mean approaching the view of the other or vindicating one's own. In the silence that surrounds any conversation, not just those created by a Beckett or a Pinter, the same line may as well be an act of hiding, as of trying to get in touch. Communication is an option and a limitation. There is usually some work to be done to create the common ground where at least two minds, each with its particular outlook, relate to the very same 'cut' of reality. But even common ground is relative. In lifelong and developing relationships, it is internalised; both parties are, in a definite sense, the common. In the shorter term, such as that of a consultation, common ground is common enough ground. It is not just the facts but also an effort that opens for a winning imperfection. What two people share is not the absolute opposite of the solipsistic isolation, which would be the free confluence of minds, but a third version. In fact, there is here something to learn from the categorical standpoint of solipsism. If it ever were a valid description of the status of mind, it would have to be generally valid. If the isolation of mind could ever be overcome, then there was not isolation from the beginning. And this must be our conclusion. Subjectivity has an open aspect in its very essence,[2] lending itself to, and reaching toward, the mutual and public. Therefore, when looking at clinical communication, looking at the real rather than the ideal makes sense. Words are not enough. What really matters is their references in real life.

SCIENTIFIC PERSPECTIVES
Evolution
Empathetic understanding is not unique to humans. Apes have a well developed emotional interplay, strengthening the life of the group. Survival of the fittest does not hold for individuals as much as for the group.[3] Even lower animals make social compromises to share the powers and security of the community. The leaps in the development of intelligence and, proportionate to that, the

enlargement of the brain seen in primates, are thought to reflect the complexity of social being. Sociality is a strong strand in evolution.

The newborn infant as communicator

Infants show communicating abilities from the very start,[4] preparing them to recognise a world containing other subjects. If this were not the case, a baby would hardly be able to imitate the behaviours of others less than an hour after birth.[5] This puts Kant's understanding of *a priori* into the concrete. In his philosophy, the *a priori* are the subjective and necessary prerequisites for experiencing the world.[6,7] Space and time are necessary to make up a comprehensive reality from the impressions from the outside world, but as forms of sensibility they do not themselves belong to reality. *A priori* in Kant's sense belongs to the idealist heritage in philosophy. It brings out 'the thing' by concealing 'the thing in itself' under the veils of subjectivity. Still, the observations referred to above seem to demonstrate the *a priori* as a biologically given faculty to become involved in the world without having experienced it before. If this conclusion is correct, then the *a priori* is intersubjective, either as an aspect of it, or as its very essence.

The mirror neurons

Apes and humans have neurons in their premotor cortex which become activated both on executing actions, and when observing the same actions executed by others.[8,9] In the latter situation, the observer gets the neurophysiological imprint of the actor's behaviour as quickly as if it were his/her own. There is no time for inferences or judgements to be made. The brains are 'paired',[10] and thus the action is immediately recognised. Movement in isolation is not enough to make the mirror neurons become active. It has to be driven by a goal; that which really makes it an action.

In addition to this, in humans there is experimental evidence for the view that groups of mirror neurons have a number of specific functions. Distinct groups of mirror neurons are involved in imitation[11] and in the recognition of mimicry and gestures. It has been suggested that this faculty represents 'the basic mechanism from which language evolved'.[12] Similar movements are 'mirrored' differently depending on context.[13] The interpretation of this observation is that the mirror neurons bear the correlate of grasping the intention of the action in a deeper sense than its mere goal. Specific mirror neurons are at work in the recognition of sensations (pain) and emotions of others.[14,15] In analogy with action understanding, it has been proposed that the grasping of emotions is mediated through the activation of mirror neurons within viscero-motor circuits.[16]

The operation of mirror neurons thus gives a biological clue to intersubjectivity and empathy. As metaphors, the magnetic resonance images of the activated clusters of neurons are quite strong, and accordingly we may anticipate an increasing interest in empathy in medicine. Obviously, what is shown in these images is not understanding in itself. The 'hard problem of consciousness', the explanatory gap between consciousness and nature,[17] has not been solved, and will most probably not be. Experience is only to be understood as experience. However, experience and scientific explanations are two versions of one and the same reality.

INTERPRETATION AND EMPATHY

Hermeneutics

For many years philosophy dealt mainly with logic, metaphysics and ethics, paying less attention to understanding as such. The appearance of hermeneutics as a distinct philosophical activity in the early 19th century expanded the boundaries. Friedrich Schleiermacher, priest and philosopher, was the pioneering figure who assembled and developed the thoughts of his contemporaries among the German romantic philosophers[18,19] into a general theory of understanding. The aim of hermeneutics was to reach an understanding of the text that was faithful to its author's thinking, intentions and context. The initial focus was on historical and religious texts. A text speaks, and hermeneutics is, according to Schleiermacher, 'the art of hearing'. Hermeneutics has become an important element in contemporary philosophy, and the basic idea that the understanding of a text comes through dialogue and not merely through analysis, is still strongly alive. According to Schleiermacher, any interpretation has two sides; the first is the agreed meaning of words (a matter of linguistics), and the second is about what the particular author actually has in his or her mind (a matter of psychology). The first side is comparative in that it builds on the reader's understanding and experiences of the references of the words; the second requires conjecture and imagination, which are essential to approach the perspective of the writer as a living and unique person. The interpretation is neither merely reproducing what is already known, nor independent of shared facts. Interpretation is also a holistic activity. What Schleiermacher introduces here is the so-called 'hermeneutic circle', a circle often referred to in humanistic research. It is only possible to understand a text as a whole. It may be the last few sentences that give the first their full meaning. At the same time, it is the parts that make up the whole, so it is not possible to grasp the whole unless you understand the parts. This is logically a paradox, which underlines the fact that interpretation goes beyond logic and the references of single words. One has to make the circle 'parts-whole-parts' several times to reach a coherent and well founded version of understanding. In a wider circle, the whole text ought to be looked at in the perspective of its own context, such as the full production of the author, the language tradition, the genre and the historical situation.

Einfühlung

Closely linked to the development of hermeneutics is the recognition of the process of 'feeling oneself into' (sich einfühlen) or related wordings. This process was expressed in various contexts of interpretation – texts, aesthetics, mental state of other persons – from the late 18th century onwards.[20,21] It was not given explicit theoretical attention, but was presumed as the possibility of adopting the outlook of other subjects. Once the specific term 'Einfühlung' was coined in 1873, this opened the way for a more active and specific exploration. Theodor Lipps claimed that people have a natural instinct to imitate the expressions of others and from that, to reach a sharing of mental states. Also, by way of Einfühlung, the beholder may overcome the absolute separation between oneself and a piece of art, and thereby grasp the intention of the artist. Imitation of postures and actions depicted in, for instance, a painting may contribute to experiencing it from 'inside'. Wilhelm Dilthey regarded Einfühlung to be the highest form of understanding, distinct from the understanding based on the commonalities of a shared world and language.[22,23] For Dilthey, Einfühlung may be obtained only through art and literature, in that it implied a re-creation of the experiences and intentions of persons created by an author or artist. This re-creation of the beholder makes the hermeneutic circle complete. Dilthey's perspective was also historical. Where art expands lived experience through fiction, history accomplishes this through a structural approach. Individuals cooperate by submitting to common agreements and goods, and the modes and structures which this cooperation produces constitute history. Subjects form history and history forms them. The structures of history do not emerge automatically by the assembling of facts. Like Einfühlung on the individual level, historical interpretation implies a imaginative effort, which makes the distinction between the two levels graded rather than categorical.

It was only in 1908 that Einfühlung was translated, by the psychologist Edward Titchener, into English through the Greek neologism 'empathy'. In the 20th century, empathy became a vital concept within phenomenology and psychology. In most of the early versions, Einfühlung/empathy was about understanding all aspects of the inner life of other subjects. For instance, Dilthey addressed thought, feeling and will. In its development within psychology, and from its extension into the medical context, there has been a strong emphasis on emotions, which in relation to its origin is a limitation.

PHENOMENOLOGY AND EMPATHY

The phenomenological approach

The core of phenomenology is the injunction of its founder, Edmund Husserl, to go 'to the things themselves'.[24–27] By this he meant a reflection on experience, in which preconceptions and theories about the objects of reality are put aside in order to discern how they really are encountered as phenomena. The closest one can get to the world is in the experience of it. Consciousness is itself directed. Consciousness does not precede its contents; it is always about something. This directedness is called intentionality, which is separate from the intentions that formulate the will. The mission Husserl had set himself was to establish a basis for scientific reasoning. In his time, around 1900, theories characterised by a speculative naturalism dominated philosophy, subordinating it to the level of other scientific disciplines. For example, the understanding of knowledge was thought to be inferred from the 'laws' of psychology, or, as the next step, from insights into brain anatomy and processes. Recent progress in the science of mind – see the section on mirror neurons – has awoken a similar materialist hope within the biomedical culture. With experience and philosophy dethroned and unlinked, it was impossible to go to the source of knowledge in a non-prejudiced way.

The pretension of Husserl that phenomenology could ground science in general has proved unrealistic. Valid knowledge about the world has increased dramatically without consulting Husserl's writings. However, as a scholarly and systematic approach to the analysis of various fields of experience on the premises of experience itself, phenomenology is a productive and practically oriented branch of philosophy. Its increasing contribution to the science of mind is just one of several illustrations of its utility.

The phenomenology of empathy

According to a fairly recent definition, empathy is a 'meta-affective cognitive capacity for grasping another's point of view'.[28] Trying to grasp the patient's point of view is the first step that must be taken by any doctor faced with any symptom presentation. In fact, this is a demonstration of how the humanities work within medicine; not as an addition but as a prerequisite and starting point. As a concept, 'humanities in medicine' is as much an insight as an ambition.

In 1917, which was quite early in the development of phenomenology, Edith Stein presented an analysis of empathy in her thesis 'On the problem of empathy'.[29] Although Edith Stein is not the only thinker in the phenomenological tradition who has written about empathy, her work stands out as comprehensive and clear, and its major insights have not been contradicted by the passing of time. In addition, it goes further than 'to the things themselves', in that Stein discovers, in the empathetic stance, the 'person' and hence moves from logic to ethics. 'On the problem of empathy' is a natural choice of text that, in giving a phenomenological perspective on empathy,[30] should help us improve our understanding of clinical communication.

Before 1917, empathy had been defined in rather general terms, both regarding its contents – the point of view of the other – and regarding what kind of knowing empathy represents. Stein's outlook is that the other is, beyond doubt, an experiencing person like myself. We share the moment and the immediate and concrete context. If I am sitting alone in a room, and then somebody else comes in, the room is no longer the same. It is not just the appearance of a new object. Neither is it just a body. It is an animated body; a person, whose actions and expressions are immediately given to me. There is somebody who knows that I am there as well, and whom I am aware is aware that I am aware of his or her presence as an experiencing person. There is attention, and there is relation before knowing anything other than the presence itself. I am pulled into this relation. The relation cannot be excluded. My choices are restricted to those about how to relate. I have to take a stand and in the early stages of an encounter, the context of which is not preset, this stand is not calculated. The stand is more about one's way of discovering and approaching the other. The 'we' is neither a guess nor a plain extrapolation from the 'I'. Thus the other is quite a specific phenomenon, and within this, her or his experience.

On the level of intersubjectivity, at first glance, I may be well aware of the most salient features of the inner life of the other. Emotion may be written in the face, and in the total bodily expression of the other. In a second step, I may imaginatively approach the point of view – 'step into the shoes' – of the other. Here my awareness shifts from what the other's experience is for me to what it means for the other. This is the 'feeling in' of Einfühlung. If it succeeds to any substantial degree, on the deepest level of intersubjectivity, I will stand beside the other, sharing the perspective. I will then realise that what the other experiences is not just any sadness, but with a shade of experienced meaninglessness, or not just any fatigue, but fatigue of a very physical kind. Stein means, that in the second, crucial step, I have no choice if I want to get to know the predicament of the other. I may choose the depth, but not the direction. I inevitably become involved in the experience of the other. In the empathetic process, therefore, the primarily experienced object which is the apprehended inner state of the other, is, at the same time, a guide into the context of the other's experience.

Empathy is not the merging of experiences. If there is no clear distinction between the other's experience and mine, then it is mine. Empathy is primarily about the other.

Stein refutes the conception that empathy relies on inference, either by association/simulation, or by mere analogy. In the first case, I see the behaviour of the other, and recognise that when I act, or look, similarly, then I usually feel in a certain way. From this I conclude that this is the way the other feels, too. In the second case, in the science of mind also known as 'theory-theory', I build my judgement cognitively on relations between cause – mental state – and effect – behaviour.

Theories of simulation[31] and analogy[32] belong to the contemporary debate in cognitive science. Taking Stein's standpoint, they bear the legacy of solipsism. She says that any inferences or conclusions about the other presuppose a primary recognition of his or her subjectivity and this recognition is in itself intersubjective. It is not a judgement from the outside but recognition from within the relation. The space between two people is always in some respect shared. The increasing insights into the immediate linking of minds through mirror neurons lend support to Stein's understanding of empathy. This linkage is what people take for granted when sharing their experiences.

Neither do psychoanalytical explanations of empathy, i.e. projection and resonance,[33,34] find support in Stein's phenomenological analysis. Empathy is not blind affect. Laughter may irresistibly spread in a group of people where very few, in fact, know what the laughter is about. Its sources are then above all idiosyncratic.

According to Stein, empathy is an act of experiencing *sui generis*. It cannot fall back on any other acts of experiencing. She makes the comparison with memory. Memory is about the past; something that is only indirectly given in consciousness, but the act of memorising is directly given. It is what being conscious is about at the moment of memorising. In a similar fashion, my awareness of what the other is experiencing is indirectly given in his or her total expression within our communication. But still, as is the case for memories, this does not make it a piece of knowledge. It is, in fact, experience, and in that sense she holds empathy, like memory, to be the direct experiencing of something that is indirectly given.

From the general to the individual

On experiential and logical grounds, Stein sees empathy as the only path for communicating experience between any two persons. It is a general claim. It has yet to be made concrete how the other, in real life encounters, steps forward as somebody whose experience can be shared. The very basic condition is the presence of the body of the other. As already pointed at, this body is animated and alive (Leib as opposite to Körper in German). It is a person, whose soul is expressed through the body. The body-soul separation is reconciled in the very appearance of the other. Tied to the animated body is the other's *field of sensation*. Through the body and its faculties a person stretches out for the world with all the available senses and with an emotional drive. Empathy could not be reserved for a single strand within this whole, where feelings are loaded with perceptions and born by cognition, and cognition is loaded with feeling and tied to perceptions. Seeing the other's hand is seeing a person's hand, and through that approaching his or her field of sensation from the point of view of the hand; sensing, working, greeting and so on.

Meeting other people reveals *other centres of orientation* in the world. Empathetically my world expands to being a world for all and independent of me. Here is the principle of reality and the recognition of facts. On the same line I become one among many subjects which is essential for understanding myself as a psychical and physical individual. I may look at myself through the eyes of others.

The other is *expressive* of his or her experience; it may be emotions or general feelings of life such as vigour or tiredness or more distinct experiences of ill health. Expressions are not signs, they are the outer aspect of a subjective stand. The soul is visible. A look of anger is anger as long as it is not pretended, and probably it is not well pretended if it is not to some degree real. In face of the animated body, inner and outer are not a dichotomy. Again, empathy is not observation but a change of consciousness from an observing position, to one where I am pulled into the position of the other.

From the individual to the spiritual

What in a deepest sense dictates empathy as different from other kinds of experiencing is that the other, being a person, relates to the world through meaning. Looking at human beings as psycho-physical beings reduces them to a behaviourist impulse-response level. In Stein's understanding, a meaning seeking consciousness goes beyond nature and the semiotic into the spiritual. Here meaning is about values. Feelings, experienced and expressed, afford value to the comprehensible in transforming it into something only partially comprehensible. In the empathic act I and the other are by definition, and from the very start, within the realm of values. Here is the opening that establishes the relation unknowingly and then puts what becomes known into place as meaningful to the other.

In making the distinction so clear between the psycho-physical or empirical being and the person, Stein regards the latter, unchanged throughout life as a given hierarchy of valuing. 'The person' may find expression to a greater or lesser degree in action and self awareness, but as potentials at every stage he or she does not change. The psycho-physical being is the individual as actualised (realised). In empathy, I may experience the potentials of the other as given, although they are not realised, and by way of my own potentials I may grasp experiences that are out of my empirical self. Only through intersubjectivity may one reach fulfilment. Here Stein ends up very close to shifting from an 'egologic' stance to one where the subject, rather than discovering the other in the empathic act, comes into being before the face of the other. Here she is touching on the theme of the philosophy of Emmanuel Levinas.[35] Also she closes the circle from the introduction of her thesis where she makes it very clear that just meeting somebody, known or unknown, in talk or wordlessly, changes all.

The role of reference in empathy

Referring to hermeneutics, one may ask how Stein understands the referential aspect of empathy. She does not comment much on the influence of likeness between subjects, nor does she address the limitations imposed by differences. Although the empathising subject may 'experience' the hitherto inexperienced, there are obvious limits to his or her potentials. Also, there are factual aspects of subjectivity that will not be taken care of by a moral relation. Benevolence is not by definition beneficent. We will come back to the role of reference when discussing empathy in the clinic.

IMAGINATION

From Plato to Kant

Moving from the first glance at the other into his or her 'shoes' takes imagination, which thus is a vital element in empathy. Imagination is the capacity to make something new out of that which is given or expected in creating and playing with alternatives – images – mentally. In art, fictions of various degrees of realism live parallel to or, as Levinas put it, on the hither side of the world.[36] In philosophy, beside the common connotation of the word, it is regarded as a mental faculty that makes sense of experience. Imagination seems to be both rational and irrational.

Mark Johnson gives a thorough account on philosophical perspectives on imagination in his book 'The mind in the body' which inspires what I say here about imagination.[37] According to Johnson, in the Platonic tradition imagination was deemed purely irrational, apt for art, although art was considered to be a dubious practice having very little to do with the true knowledge of ideas. The romantic notion of a genius was in fact nurtured by the stern idealism of Platonism, which still resides as latent scientism in contexts where science plays an important role, as it does in medicine.

Aristotle saw it differently. His argument was that there must be something to mediate between perception and thought, something that makes the sensory representations understandable, and to him that was imagination. Imagination is the capacity of the human mind to create images, which are the inner representations of the perceived world. There is no knowledge without imagination. This idea has persisted throughout the development of philosophical thought.

Kant's view was based on the notion of empiricism that imagination stands for the capacity of the mind to 'form unified images, and to recall in memory past images, so as to constitute a unified and coherent experience.' This is necessary to make judgement, i.e. to make statements about the facts of the world. But there is more to it. From the mental processing of experience, and making a whole out of its manifold, grows the 'I' of reflection and the 'empirical self' of inner experience. There has to be an 'I' to say 'not I', to distinguish the subjective from the objective. The reflective 'I' is this edge of the knife of consciousness.[38] The appearance of the 'I' has also occupied the theorists of artificial intelligence. What is it that makes me a thinking person, rather than being that which happens to occur in my brain? What is the difference between artificial intelligence and the 'I' of intelligence?

A Kantian answer would be imagination; its 'productive' function constitutes the unity of consciousness in the single moment as well as through time.

Imagination is to Kant also the power of creative reflection. To see alternatives among defined concepts you need a free space for the comparison and judgement of them. And you need to create new alternatives where none of the available ones fit. The recognition of beauty, or creating it, is according to Kant, neither random nor subjective. There is truth in beauty, although it is not possible to tie to it any definite concept, which in his theory of judgement is what warrants objectivity. Johnson sees here a clear tension within Kant's thinking between judgements of beauty and 'the restricted framework' of other kinds of judgement.

Last, imagination is the faculty of symbolising. Something is what it is, but yet what it is not. This doubling of meaning is accomplished through the use of metaphors and references. Rather than seeing it as the highest step of the staircase of imagination, one could easily regard it as the very material of the steps. Our symbolising capacity is the precondition for making any reflection whatsoever. If there were no imagination at the foundation of thought, we would have nothing but the noise of transmitters echoing across the synaptic spaces. There would be no art, no science, just the brain talking to the brain about the brain.

A contemporary view

Mark Johnson agrees with Kant that the link between imagination and rationality is unconditional. Maybe he even ascribes more to imagination in Kant's philosophy of reason than some other thinkers would do. However, he finds Kant's perspective so highly theoretical and elaborate that there is no room for imagination to work. At the centre of his own analysis, and at the bottom of language, like the soil that makes language flourish, are originally embodied 'image schemata', and their metaphorical projections across domains of experience, in the constitution of meaning.[39] Even in our most abstract arguments, body experiences ground linguistic meaning. 'What are often thought of as abstract meanings and inferential patterns actually do depend on schemata derived from our bodily experience and problem-solving.' Logic may be seen as abstraction from relations of objects and forces in space-time. Examples of such 'image schemata' are 'container', 'balance', 'centre-periphery', and 'restraint-removal'.

Imagination and empathy

What does it mean to approach, in Edith Stein's words, the subjective position of the other imaginatively? Empathy is about the experience of reality, but what the two subjects share is a new version of the original experience of one of them. The experiencer contributes with the original experience and an invitation to be approached, the empathiser with her or his involvement, integrity, references, and imagination. Being the faculty of mind to go from sensation to lived experience, imagination is also what makes intersubjectivity work. Imagination is that certain form and degree of approximation that makes rationality play. It is faithful to the given in going beyond it. Therefore, empathy is not the cloning of experience. The slight changes of meaning, and the partial misunderstandings, belong to the real life version of understanding, but unlike solipsism, they point at the possibility of communication. They are part of the effort, and never completely gone. The intersubjective world that we agree to treat as the real one is derived from the many individual ones through empathic imagination and calibration in the process of historical and scientific development. Here, more or less globally conceived aspects of reality stand side by side with those that are idiosyncratic and those that form specific cultures and subcultures.

The imperfection of empathy, resting on imagination as it does, tells that knowledge about the world of the other may never be exhaustive. Knowledge does not found the relationship. Instead, this is taken care of by the moral blend of humility and curiosity that make people inhabit a common world.

EMPATHY IN THE CLINIC
Two depths of professional readiness

A diagnosis implies the process of finding out whether an illness experience is caused by a disease, and, if so, the nature of the disease. The diagnosis is the biomedical definition of the deviation from the normal state of the organism. To the person it often is the recognition and the explanation of that which is wrong and troubling, and as such it is a powerful forecast. In its pragmatic sense, the diagnosis directs action. When permanent, the diagnosis is an addition to the person's identity.

The rest of this chapter deals with the diagnosis as a process between doctor and patient, and as an aspect of their relationship. It is about the pivoting between experience and abstraction through the pathway of communication. Both patient and doctor experience and make abstractions, but from different outlooks, and therefore with differing content. The patient has the illness experience and makes an effort to understand and deal with it. The doctor has the experience of the symptom presentation, and makes professional abstractions of different kinds. Although the illness experience and the doctor's professional knowledge and skills form a complementary relationship, in face of the bodily-existential conditions that are the implicit themes of symptom presentations, they meet in symmetry. Therefore, a doctor has two possible depths of his/her professional readiness. One is the formal, mainly biomedical knowledge, through which the doctor knows about the patient what he or she does not know. This is taken for granted by everyone. The other depth is the lived experience of the body; the existential anatomy. Here, patient and doctor have much in common as bodily imagining and communicating selves.[40-42] In terms of empathy, the bodily existential perspective is essential, but, as we shall see, the scientific perspective is not merely one of detached observation.

The presentation of a new symptom

Whether insidious or sudden, subtle or intense, the arrival of the illness is an intrusion. Perception is changed in a negative fashion and there is a rift in the sense of normality. The existential anatomy is under change. Here, invasion, loss, or restraint are the immediate gross characteristics of symptoms that mandate attention.[43] The new situation evokes interpretations – 'the hermeneutic moment'[44] – merging intuition, experience and pieces of formal knowledge: 'Can I stand this? What may be the cause? What will happen? Is it dangerous?' Tentative lay diagnoses may line up, reassuring or frightening. At this stage, when no doctor is yet consulted, the diagnosis is eventualities and questions. When the symptom is in itself endurable, the individual's diagnostic considerations formulate the decision to seek, or not to seek, a doctor. The more severe the ailment, the more the decision is a reflex action in the search for help.

However, even when having made their own preliminary diagnoses, few patients start off the consultation by suggesting it. They usually present their symptom and the content and form of this presentation decide what the consultation will be about. It is only in the abstract that doctors assess and judge symptoms. In practice they receive and react to symptom presentations, in which the original experiences are enveloped in the patients' diagnostic considerations, their expectations and immediate needs, and their repertoire of expressions. Some examples may illustrate this:

A serious and scary symptom which is perceived as serious may be played down in the presentation in hoping that the doctor will say it is not serious.

A minor sensation may be considerably augmented by fear, the latter dominating in the presentation. A problem that has been with the patient for years, for instance low back pain, that in fact has not changed, may be presented with more impressive features once the patient, after discussing with the spouse, has decided that now is the time for a MRI scan.

Empathy and diagnosis

Finding out about the diagnosis is by necessity a strong drive in doctors. As the symptom is being presented, they are flipping through the pages of their inner symptom dictionaries[45] and therefore may listen primarily for those accounts that are suggestive of clear-cut diseases, and which carry the promise of a corresponding clarity of answers and pieces of advice. This is the biomedical reflex, an automatic response developed in medical education, and very adequate in emergencies.[46] Once the reflex position has been taken, doctors observe what is told rather than interacting with their patients. The real life situation approaches the abstraction. When the match between a hypothesis and the cues is good enough, the tentative diagnosis shows the way forward. The pace and elegance of the biomedical method, when it is working, is compelling. However, it incurs risks. The patient may feel that the doctor lacks interest in his particular situation, causing him to withdraw. Such a defect of communication may lead to shallowness, and even diagnostic misunderstandings. Many symptoms lack obvious biological correlates, and disease experiences have individual features and interpretations colouring their presentations. Also, through the patient's withdrawal much of the cooperative potential of the patient-doctor relation may be lost. The patient-centred clinical method,[47] and Pendleton's consultation model,[48] and other similar initiatives, have all been developed to restore communication and cooperation, taking the biomedical reflex for granted.

An unprejudiced approach to the symptom presentation, where the doctor tries to share the patient's experience in its own right and irrespective of its cause, may lead doctor and patient onto a common track from the very beginning. By 'common track' I mean a truly shared effort to come to an understanding of the patient's problem. It is not so much a matter of words as of how the doctor relates to the patient. It is also paying respect to the fact that the making of a diagnosis, in all those cases where this is not directly given through undisputable signs, is a two-step process. The first step is bodily empathetic. The doctor has to be let in into the world of the patient. Here body and person, as well as diagnosis and person, are one. In Stein's terminology, the doctor approaches the fields of the sensation of the patient.

In Jake's case, for instance, this is not reached primarily through a 'clinical gaze' on those parts of the body that are involved in the symptoms. Instead, the doctor imagines Jake's experience from within his predicament of being dominated by both skin and bowel irritation. In terms of neuronal activity, only a minor part of what is perceived and presented as bodily sensations stems from the specific sensory nerve ends. All the central nervous system contributes to the conscious sensation.[49] Empathy is about the immediate bodily experiences as well as about their context. Both cast light on each other and contribute to the total grasp of Jake's symptoms and the suffering they cause.

Words like tiredness, dizziness and itching do not primarily refer to symptoms. They have general meanings that we can understand because of what the words mean to us. But we also need to understand what these words mean to the person who presents them. This meaning can only be clarified in a dialogue with him or her. The doctor's own existential anatomy, sensitised through the manifold of bodily dialogues in their work, the intersubjective learning and expansion of body experience from thousands of symptom presentations and the general biomedical facts integrated into experience, give the references for the imagination. Clinical work is bodily empathic training, and if open to its opportunities, the doctor's attention becomes a sounding-board of bodily experience.

The second step of diagnosis includes biomedical detachment and judgement[50] or other objectifying stances. Rather than being chronological, the two steps are continuously interweaving like a breathing of consciousness. The accuracy of the second step is dependent on the sensitivity in the first. The recognition that neither step is dispensable enfolds patient and disease within one and the same act of attention which ultimately is of moral character.

General bodily empathy and the mental

Bodily empathy is not reserved for doctors. It is a general human capacity to empathically approach the body experiences of others, including the emotions and thoughts that are immediately attached to what is perceived. It is the process by which existential anatomy becomes intersubjectivity. It should not be thought of as one side of a dichotomy of empathy where emotional/cognitive empathy is the other. It is the field of empathy where the emphasis is the body experience. Since mind is embodied,[51] bodily empathy is an aspect also of the communication of emotions and thoughts. It is not possible to detach an emotion from its vegetative accompaniment, nor a thought from its horizons in physical reality. From the perspective of embodiment, the division between the mental and physical is an artefact. Nevertheless, at a certain moment consciousness favours either thoughts, or sensations, or emotions. A patient usually knows whether to see a surgeon or a psychiatrist.

THE DIAGNOSIS AS UNDERSTANDING: THE STORIES

To find a proper diagnosis is gratifying to any doctor. It incorporates the patient's complaints with the doctor's professional territory. It validates one's competence. Algorithms for the succeeding steps in management will usually be available. Once the biomedical step of diagnosis is complete it may therefore be tempting to stay on this level, substituting politeness for intersubjectivity and then moving on to the next patient. But as much as a diagnosis invites recognition in an observational sense, it may deepen the rapport between patient and doctor. Knowing the facts of the disease is also knowing very important things from the patient's perspective.

Rachel's young doctor brings the diagnosis of diabetes to her bedside. To Rachel the message is like a 'hard, cold bell'. Hard and cold as nature itself inside her body, and as the technical devices that stand out from the children-friendly atmosphere of the ward. The facts of the own body excludes negotiation. The character of treatment – injections that 'dig holes' in her skin, in Rachel herself – corresponds with the way the disease has invaded her life. Although she, in the cognitive sense, probably has limited understanding of what is going on, she knows a lot in a direct way. We do not know if the doctor, either informed by professional knowledge about what the diabetes diagnosis means to children or by intuition, grasps that Rachel is in such a hard, cold place. Anyway, she seems to rely a lot on Dax, the nurse. Maybe this will be OK for Rachel, but on the whole, it is not enough that a doctor only stands for the facts when there are hard facts to be given. At that moment Rachel needs someone to share the experience with, and no one could do this better than the doctor who is responsible for explaining what is happening. She is sitting beside Rachel, knows the facts, and is exposed to the immediate need of her young patient. Rachel would have been better off if her doctor had heard the metallic sound of the diagnosis. Facts and support are always indivisible in a doctor's commitment.

Jake's strongly felt unease is about exposing his behind as part of the diagnostic investigation. Originally, the danger signal, blood in the stools, was strong enough to overcome his anxiety about being examined. But once he lies before the scrutinising gaze of Dr Siddha, he is a captive of the situation itself. He does not like to expose his body at all. Usually, his skin condition holds him back, but now Dr Siddha intrudes into his bodily interior. She is correctly quite aware of Jake's embarrassment, and succeeds in making him believe that this is nothing but an everyday task for her. If behind this attitude she is a bit tense herself, this is, according Edith Stein, her own tension rather than the empathic sensing of that of Jake's. But while she is engaged in controlling her own feelings, she is not well equipped to see the situation from Jake's perspective. So maybe the recognition of her own tension is still the key to an empathic move into Jake's predicament, in which he finds himself experiencing the unimaginable. More than just tuning into Jake's emotion, empathy is here about imagining fairly concretely what the exposure means to Jake. Unfortunately, her medical jargon adds to the distance, and when she finally asks about his psoriasis Jake does not feel it is really about him. Dr Siddha is probably trying as hard as she can under the circumstances – he is, after all, her last patient in a much delayed surgery. In sensitive situations, the balance between self-control and openness is hard to strike. The significance of bodily empathy in a technical procedure like proctoscopy is, however, the continuing recognition of the dignity of the patient. To Jake, or any other patient in a similar situation, pushed into it by the merciless body, the doctor is very present. Everything is registered; the touch, the tone of voice, and the grunts or other wordless sounds that Byrne and Long called 'miscellaneous professional noises'.[52] The patient's attention is on getting these paralinguistic messages right. 'What do they tell about me?' The relation is never closed, and if the doctor tries to abdicate from it, the patient is very likely to feel dismissed. There is a request for steadiness on behalf of the doctor when life itself is so unpredictable.

While the examining gynaecologist judges the difference between a normal and a slightly abnormal pap smear to be quite small, it is for Liz a gulf between life and death. But Liz is lucky; her doctor is not stuck with the cytological estimates. Over the phone, and very quickly, she imagines Liz standing in the airport with her daughter waiting, overwhelmed by fear and just about to miss the flight. The doctor is also well aware of Liz's sensitivity and insecurity and seems to feel a parallel between the present situation and Liz's epileptic fit at an earlier examination: thrown into the world, lonely and confused, and with an unreliable body. Where she is now, her daughter cannot distract her. The only one who can rescue their holiday is the doctor, and this is what she does.

Jen looks at her doctor in the thoracic department with sympathy, but not really at him as a doctor. From her point of view, the person and the doctor take on very different roles. She also seems to hear what Dr Murray says from a certain distance. Memories, associations, and conclusions work inside her head. She is only partly there. Her greatest dread is TB. The shadow on the X-ray is a forecast of the fate that killed her mother and hit her brother. Then comes the word 'cancer' and the question about smoking, and the regret over all the years of smoking without even enjoying it. Meaninglessness and confusion is what she feels on her way home. The bus ride in the dark city turns into a passage to the kingdom of the dead. The doctor did never recognise what was going on. The only hint was Jen's question about TB, but beside that she gave him few chances. We know nothing about Dr Murray apart from what he said, and that he, in Jen's eyes, looked sympathetic. We do not know whether his anonymity was due to the fact that Jen was unable to respond to him and therefore deaf to invitations to talk about her personal reaction to the probable diagnosis. It may be very difficult for a doctor to approach the patient in a bodily empathic sense, when he or she hides behind an apparently compliant face. It is not likely that communication was confused because Dr Murray limited his role to delivering 'disease medicine' only. Any doctor would know that when cancer is the possible disease, the issue from the point of view of the patient is as much death as it is cancer.

Dr Gaitens knows Geoff quite well, as well as he knows his wife Jen, who is now in hospital. When he steps into the bedroom, he sees it all at once; the stroke-ridden and bitter man, now hit even harder by the painful absence of his ever-loving wife. Depression is his whole expression. It is sculpted into his shrinking, stubborn and dry body. He says no to everything. Here is no division of body and soul. Here is just suffering.

REFERENCES
1 Russell B. *History of Western Philosophy*. London: Routledge; 2004, pp. 589–99.
2 Thompson E, Zahavi D. Philosophical issues: Phenomenology. In: Zelazo PD, Moscovitch M, Thompson E, editors. *The Cambridge Handbook of Consciousness*. Cambridge: Cambridge University Press; 2007.

3 De Waal F, Thompson E. Interviewed by Jim Proctor: Primates, Monks, and the Mind. The Case of Empathy. *Journal of Consciousness Studies*. 2005; **12**: 38–54.

4 Trevarthen C. Facial expressions of emotion in mother-infant interaction. *Human Neurobiology*. 1985; **4**: 21–32.

5 Meltzoff AN, Moore MK. Newborn infants imitate adult facial gestures. *Child Development*. 1983; **54**: 702–9.

6 Russell B, op. cit., pp. 637–51.

7 Hanna R. Kant's Theory of Judgment. In: *Stanford Encyclopedia of Philosophy*. http://plato.stanford.edu/entries/kant-judgment/

8 Rizzolatti G. The mirror neuron system and its functions in humans. *Anatomy and Embryology*. 2005; **210**: 419–21.

9 Gallese V. The 'shared manifold' hypothesis. From mirror neurons to empathy. *Journal of Consciousness Studies*. 2001; **8**: 33–50.

10 Thompson E. Empathy and consciousness. *Journal of Consciousness Studies*. 2001; 8(5–7): 1–32.

11 Rizzolatti, op. cit.

12 Rizzolatti G, Arbib MA. Language within our grasp. *Trends in Neurosciences*. 1998; **21**: 188–94.

13 Iacobini M, Molnar-Szakacs, Gallese V *et al.* Grasping the intentions of others with one's own mirror neuron system. *PLoS Biology*. 2005; 3(3): 529–35.

14 Gallese, op. cit.

15 Rizzolatti, op. cit.

16 Gallese V, Keysers C, Rizzolatti G. A unifying view on the basis of social cognition. *Trends in Cognitive Sciences*. 2004; **8**: 396–403.

17 Thompson, op. cit.

18 Palmer RE. *Hermeneutics*. Evanston, IL: Northwestern University Press; 1969, pp. 84–97.

19 Forster M. Friedrich Daniel Ernst Schleiermacher. In: *Stanford Encyclopedia of Philosophy*. http://plato.stanford.edu/entries/schleiermacher/

20 Nilsson P. *Empathy and Emotions. On the notion of empathy as emotional sharing*. Umeå: Umeå Studies in Philosophy; 2003, pp. 67–73.

21 Stueber K. Empathy. In: *The Stanford Encyclopedia of Philosophy*. http://plato.stanford.edu/entries/empathy/index.html

22 Makkreel R, Dilthey W. In: *The Stanford Encyclopedia of Philosophy*. http://plato.stanford.edu/entries/dilthey/

23 Palmer, op. cit., pp. 98–123.

24 Thompson, Zahavi, op. cit.

25 Karlsson G. *Psychological Qualitative Research from a Phenomenological Perspective*. Stockholm: Almqvist & Wiksell International; 1995, pp. 43–55.

26 Toombs K. Introduction: Phenomenology and Medicine. In: Toombs K, editor. *Handbook of Phenomenology and Medicine*. Dordrecht: Kluwer Academic Publishers; 2001.

27 Husserl E. *The Crisis of European Sciences and Transcendental Phenomenology*. Evanston, IL: Northwestern University Press; 1970.

28 Thompson, op. cit.

29 Stein E. *On the Problem of Empathy*. Washington, DC: ICS Publications; 1989.

30 These comments on 'On the problem of empathy' are indebted to the Norwegian

philosopher Magdalene Thomassen, who has published a 'near reading' of Stein's text in an anthology published in Norwegian about the life and writings of Edith Stein. Möller M, Nygård M. *Edith Stein. Filosof och mystiker.* Oslo: Emilia; 2000, pp. 96–146.

31 Goldman AI. Folkpsychology and mental concepts. *Protosociology.* 2000; **14**: 4–25.

32 Gopnik A. How we know our minds. The illusion of first-person knowledge of intentionality. *Behavioural and Brain Sciences.* 1993; **16**: 1–14.

33 Buie D. Empathy: Its nature and limitations. *Journal of American Psychoanalytical Association.* 1981; **29**: 281–307.

34 Basch MF. Empathic understanding. A review of the concept and some theoretical considerations. *Journal of American Psychoanalytical Association.* 1983; **31**: 101–26.

35 Thomassen M. The other – the face of infinity. The transcendence philosophy of Emmanuel Levinas. (Norwegian title: Den andre – uendelighetens ansikt). In: H Koslstad, H Bjornstad, A Aarnes, editors. *Tracing Infinity. A book of discussion on Emmanuel Levinas.* (Norwegian title: *I sporet av det uendelige. En debattbok om Emmanuel Levinas*). Oslo: Aschehoug; 1995, pp. 47–76.

36 Levinas E. La réalité et son ombre. *Les temps moderne.* 1948; **4**: 771–89. Norwegian translation: Aarnes A. Virkeligheten och dess skygge. In: *Underveis mot den annen. Essäer av och om Levinas.* Oslo: Vidarforlaget; 1998, pp. 13–30.

37 Johnson M. *The Mind in the Body – The Bodily Basis of Meaning, Imagination and Reason.* London: University of Chicago Press; 1988, pp. 147–66.

38 Brook A. Kant's view of the mind and consciousness of self. In: *Stanford Encyclopedia of Philosophy.* http://plato.stanford.edu/entries/kant-mind/

39 Johnson, op. cit., pp. 63–138 and 166–72.

40 Cassell EJ. *Clinical Technique, Vol. 2, Talking With Patients.* Cambridge, MA: MIT Press; 1985.

41 Engel G. Commentary on Schwarz and Wiggins: Science, humanism, and the nature of medical practice. *Perspectives in Biology and Medicine.* 1985; **28**: 362–5.

42 Rudebeck CE. General practice and the dialogue of clinical practice: on symptoms, symptom presentations and bodily empathy. *Scand J Prim Health Care.* 1992; **Suppl 1**: 79–80.

43 Rudebeck CE. The body as lived experience in health and disease. In: M Evans, R Ahlzén, I Heath, J Macnaughton, editors. *Medical Humanities Companion. Volume 1 Symptom.* Oxford: Radcliffe Publishing; 2008.

44 Leder D. *The Absent Body.* Chicago, IL: Chicago University Press; 1990, p. 78.

45 Barrows AS, Norman GR, Neufeld VR, Feightner JW. The clinical reasoning of randomly selected physicians in general medical practice. *Clinical and Investigative Medicine.* 1982; **5**: 49–55.

46 Rudebeck CE. The doctor, the patient and the body. *Scand J Prim Health Care.* 2000; **18**: 4–8.

47 Stewart M, Belle Brown J, McWhinney IR *et al. Patient Centred Medicine.* London: Sage Publications; 1995.

48 Pendleton D, Schofield T, Tate P, Havelock P. *The Consultation. An approach to teaching and learning.* London: Oxford University Press; 1984.

49 Varela FJ, Thompson E, Rosch E. *The Embodied Mind. Cognitive science and human experience.* London: MIT Press; 1991.

50 McWhinney IR. Being a general practitioner: what it means. *Euro J Gen Prac.* 2000; **6**: 135–9.
51 Thompson, op. cit.
52 Byrne PS, Long BEL. *Doctors Talking to Patients.* Exeter: Royal College of General Practitioners; 1976.

CHAPTER 9

A diagnostic jungle? Ambiguities in classification

JYRKI KORKEILA

A patient complains about recurrent unwelcome thoughts that are causing him distress. He fears that he might accidentally carry out some of the violent acts that he is unable to resist thinking about. After the interview, he is relieved to know that his condition is called obsessive-compulsive disorder: 'So, these thoughts do not mean that I am really bad, deep down?' he says.

How does a psychiatric diagnosis function? First, it may give reassurance that one is not alone in an experience and that a doctor may be able to help. Second, a diagnosis may function to distance the sufferer from a distressing experience. A patient may then feel 'this is not my fault; this condition is neither deliberate nor self-imposed'. One of the most effective psychotherapies for depression uses a perspective that enables patients to feel less guilty; the assignment of the sick role is one of the cornerstones of interpersonal psychotherapy.

However, this does not mean that a diagnosis removes all personal responsibility. We still see individuals as morally culpable if they commit violent acts, knowing them to be harmful, and we still expect patients with an addiction to make moral choices about their future behaviour if they expect help from others.

Rachel wants to know 'Am I a diabetic?' The answer to this question has implications for life and identity. A psychiatric disorder alters a patient's self-concept even more profoundly than an organic disorder. According to sociologist Richard Sennet, our self-respect is based on feeling respected as a member of society and as a person able to give something of value to others.[1] A patient with schizophrenia may simply want someone to trust him enough to give him a job. He has two burdens: the illness itself and the associated stigma. The fate of the person with schizophrenia is likely to fall short of a sense of agency. Society's attitudes towards schizophrenia shed light on our deepest values and fears, and especially our difficulties in dealing with the frailty of the human condition.

WHAT ARE DIAGNOSES AND WHAT ARE DISEASES?

Diagnoses can describe pathology, suggest aetiology, guide treatment and provide information on prognosis. Diagnoses can also promote communication between health professionals, facilitate follow-up of patient groups and guide resource allocation.

'Disease', 'disorder' and 'medical condition' are often used interchangeably. Diseases can be defined as deviations from the norm (in the statistical-biological sense), social constructions or subjective accounts of the general state of persons. The definitions of disease in five different standard dictionaries differ to an extent that indicates that the term 'disease' does not carry a precise meaning. 'The definitions do not permit an easy decision about what to include under the category and what to exclude.'[2]

Illnesses on the other hand are essentially experiential, and psychiatric illnesses present a special case because they may appear to be entirely experiential, lacking any identifiable anatomical or physiological pathology.

No matter how hard we try to remove them, the concept of disease 'cannot be used without value-judgements slipping back in'.[3] There is a difference between recognising what is *judged* to be a disease in a particular culture (but not in another culture) and stating what *is* a disease under any circumstances. The search for the unchanging essence of a disease may not be very helpful, because the concept itself is liable to change as medical knowledge increases. General definitions of disease must always leave room for disagreement on whether to include a condition as disease or not, and will inevitably fail to take into consideration new knowledge or special circumstances.[4]

Alternatively, diseases and disorders could be defined in terms of what needs to be done to restore a patient to health. Disease would then signify the potential to benefit from treatment or care. On this basis, the definition of mental illness might read as follows:

> Something is a (mental illness) if and only if it is an abnormal and involuntary process that does (mental) harm and should best be treated by medical[5] means.[6]

According to Fulford[7] the philosophical issues related to medicine as a whole are more conspicuous in psychiatry, but the core issues remain in any branch of medical care. Kendler[8] has argued that psychiatry is 'particularly susceptible to preconceptions that can strongly colour the value we assign to methodological perspectives' because psychiatry deals with fundamental questions of what it means to be human. We describe and define anxiety in more ways than juvenile diabetes or psoriasis. The personal significance of diabetes or psoriasis is easier to outline than that of social anxiety disorder or conduct disorder. The latter two raise distinctive questions of a social and political nature: how should one behave and how far can one stray before being considered pathological?

The fact that a disease or disorder is value-laden does not mean that it cannot be studied as an object of scientific inquiry. It is rather a question of *how* values matter. Medicine and psychiatry require philosophical, ethical and ecological sensibility. Even in cases where relatively objective, opinion-free information is available, issues of values accompany every patient who steps into the doctor's office.

WHY CLASSIFICATION?

Classification is basic to human cognition.

> Without the ability to categorise, we could not function at all, either in the physical world or in our social and intellectual lives. An understanding of how we categorise is central to any understanding of how we think and how we function, and therefore central to an understanding of what makes us human.[9]

A classification of psychiatric disorders provides a common language between the professionals; a classification system guides information retrieval. 'Syndromes' become important because some symptoms tend to cluster in particular ways. The modern classification systems, the Diagnostic Statistical

Manual (DSM) and International Classification of Diseases (ICD), describe these syndromes with certain, defined patterns as diagnostic categories. It is important to highlight here that the diagnoses *do not* describe the person who suffers from the condition.

A diagnostic classification should provide tools for choice of treatments and information on prognosis. Furthermore, the classification system creates a conceptual basis for scientific research. Blasfield and Burgess state that 'control of the classification system affects the models of research that make sense for mental health funding by both government and the private sector. It also has strong influence on the types of decisions that mental health professionals make'.[10] A classification system may fulfil these aims in different ways at different times. It may meet the requirements of each particular aspect to a varying extent.

'HOUSTON, WE HAVE A PROBLEM!'

Currently, there are more than 300 categories in the DSM-IV-TR classification, but this figure does not represent the actual number of disorders, because subcategories describe the severity of symptoms or phase of illness. Historically, psychiatry has waxed and waned between 'lumping' and 'splitting'. In addition to classifying disorders into a few large or many small groups, there is also the question of whether psychiatry should be classified as part of the natural sciences or the human sciences. The development of technology and the methods of neuroscience have given a strong impetus toward the current view of psychiatry as a science. Neuroscientific research has and will continue to enhance psychiatry positively, As a result, perhaps the humanistic view and the subjective realm have been downsized.

The current approach promotes a narrow view of psychopathology and what is important in a clinical context. If not understood as a useful tool, classifications can influence clinicians to pay attention to features defined within the disease criteria. Moreover, patients do have many other concerns that may need to be addressed in the clinical encounter. For a person with major depression, interpersonal trouble may be the presenting problem and depression may be the cause or result. It may be useful to remember that, although illnesses and disorders can be identified by a set of defined characteristics in a patient, they have no independent existence. Diagnoses may have high utility among professionals, but their utility is low in the lives of most patients, some of whom have negative experiences of diagnostic labelling.

Zachar[11] has argued that mental disorders are not natural categories definable with reference to inherent properties that are 'natural things in nature'. Instead of natural kinds, Zachar suggests the use of a concept of 'practical kinds'. These are stable patterns that can be identified with varying levels of reliability and validity. Fuzzy borders mean that we cannot always tell whether a phenomenon belongs to one category or not. Psychiatric diagnoses are necessarily arbitrary in certain respects, but that does not make them unreliable or invalid.

DYSFUNCTION AS THE PASSWORD TO DISORDER

The DSM formulation of disorder as 'clinically significant dysfunction that limits personal freedom and increases risk of death' is an attempt to apply values that are universally appreciated.[12] 'Antisocial personality disorder' is a label that should only be applied to an individual whose behaviour is harmfully dysfunctional.

Two important theoretical models define mental disorders from the functional viewpoint. These models cover both objective and evaluative domains and have the potential to serve as foundations for an integrative science of psychiatry. According to Wakefield,[13] mental disorders should be defined as harmful failures of internal mechanisms to perform their naturally selected functions. This view rejects both consideration of disorder as merely a value concept that refers to harmful external conditions (illness as mere social malaise) and disorder as a purely medical-scientific concept. Rather, the concept of harmful dysfunction suggests that the diagnosis of a mental disorder requires both a scientific judgement of an actual failure and a value judgement that the failure harms the individual. A disorder cannot be identified unless there are negative consequences for evolutionary adaptiveness, e.g. capacity to reproduce and to take care of oneself and one's family. Wakefield's view has been challenged on the grounds that some mental functions may be evolutionary by-products rather than results of adaptation.[14]

In an Aristotelian view on the concept of mental disorder, illness is defined as an 'incapacitating failure of a human to act as it must if the agent as a whole is to live a fully rational life'.[15] Rational here signifies 'a good life' that is essentially social in its nature, as man is a political animal. Moreover, rational life means among other things behaviour that is optimal for the persistence of the species. Health could thus be defined by analysing the fundamental nature of the 'good life'. Mental illnesses incapacitate rational functioning by a direct attack on the agent's rational powers. This prevents him/her from forming rational beliefs on the basis of information or making choices in the light of desires and beliefs. In the Aristotelian natural world, facts and values are necessarily fused; evaluative accounts of functions are also factual accounts. The distinction between vice and illness is that one condition is within one's power to change, but the other is not.[16]

SOME AMBIGUITIES IN PSYCHIATRIC DIAGNOSIS

Sadler[17] has identified five types of contextual background. Psychiatric syndromes are more ambiguous than physical illnesses regarding the questions 'did I make the illness?' or 'is the illness something that simply happened to me?' In all of the narratives belonging to Rachel, Jake and the others, illness interfered with their lives while they were busy making other plans. Illness or even mere fear of illness can be distressing. No doubt one essential feature of illnesses in these narratives is that illness manifests as something threatening one's personal control; one must decide whether to 'fight' or 'surrender'. A psychiatric disorder may impair the sense of ownership of experience or agency that provides the ability to solve the problems associated with the condition; a psychotic person perceives that the voices in his head are caused by an evil neighbour. Sometimes, in so-called dissociative states, an individual may feel that the world is distant and unreal. The self is in the foreground in psychiatry and the treatments that are available may alter the way one thinks, feels and acts. Sometimes a patient feels ambivalent about medication – or psychotherapy for that matter – due to fear of changing into a different person. A disorder may be an asset or liability, impairment or inspiration, and even the subject of moral judgements by others. A diagnosis of attention deficit-hyperactivity disorder (ADHD) may be more desirable and less stigmatising than antisocial personality disorder or simply being 'in a mess'. One diagnosis may signify hope and the other hopelessness. Lastly, Sadler lists psychiatry's social power as a source of ambiguity, since psychiatrists have the power to commit their patients into hospitals.

Proponents of 'anti-diagnosis' often call for a more holistic view of man, but they paint a picture of psychiatric diagnosis that tends to be simplistic and reductionist. Criticisms of psychiatric diagnosis usually concentrate on one aspect of psychiatric care and omit others. The aim of psychiatry is not to coerce patients, but to alleviate suffering. Any critique based on social control needs to be considered from the perspective of an ethical cost-benefit analysis for the patient himself or herself.[18]

It seems that the anti-diagnostician's paradigmatic disease is a value-neutral concept that is definable in terms of biology. Schizophrenia becomes a physical illness once the precise brain pathology is identified. The anti-diagnostician argues that mental phenomena are in the realm of meaning, and therefore mental illnesses cannot exist, because meanings cannot be ill. While this is true, the argument itself comes very close to claiming that mental phenomena do not themselves involve brain functions.

SETTING DIAGNOSES IN PRACTICE

Diagnosis discloses what may not usually be evident to the patient. Diagnosis may be seen as a tool for understanding experiences that may feel strange and incomprehensible. Diagnosis is purposeful knowledge with the ultimate aim of alleviating suffering. Making a diagnosis – and defining the criteria by which the diagnosis is made – is a privilege for physicians who are obligated by laws and authorities not to misuse their privileges. The diagnostic process is both rational in the sense that it has to rely on phenomena that can be confirmed by other clinicians, and ritual in the sense that there are commonly agreed, faithfully practised and rigorous methods to gather information required for diagnosis.[19]

Diagnoses must be valid and reliable, but they must also be useful in everyday clinical practice. Concepts with high utility tend to be easy to grasp; this was put succinctly by Lakoff and Johnson: 'It is easy to imagine a car, but more difficult to imagine what a vehicle is.'[20]

LASTLY

Psychiatric illnesses are defined in relation to the dysfunction and distress that they cause, a conceptualisation that is shared by diagnosticians and anti-diagnosticians alike. Nancy Andreasen, a biological psychiatrist and the author of *Broken Brain*, has stated that progress in neuroscience merely underlines the importance of the medical humanities, and especially the conceptual issues that occur within psychiatry as a science.

As the stories clearly show, Rachel, Jake, Liz, Geoff and Jen all experience psychological reactions to their illness experience. It is essential to find out what they value, and how their values relate to one another. Equally important is the task of understanding how the physician's values relate to individual patients' values and how they compare with those held by the profession as a whole.

If sensitivity to values is not taken seriously in clinical practice and in medical education, alienation among patients, their relatives and the population at large will increase. Modern day healthcare has become an industrial activity and the technology-zeitgeist threatens one of the most precious and fragile aspects of the doctor-patient relationship, the mutual recognition and negotiation of values.

REFERENCES

1 Sennet R. *Respect: The formation of character in an age of inequality*. London: Penguin Books; 2003.
2 Guze S. *Why Psychiatry is a Branch of Medicine*. New York: Oxford University Press; 1992.
3 Fulford KWM. Analytic philosophy, brain science and the concept of disorder. In: S Bloch, P Chodoff, SA Green, editors. *Psychiatric Ethics*. 3rd ed. Oxford: Oxford University Press; 1999.
4 Guze, op. cit.
5 Medical also comprises here psychotherapeutic treatments.
6 Reznek L. *The Philosophical Defense of Psychiatry*. New York: Routledge; 1991.
7 Fulford, op. cit.
8 Kendler KS. Toward a philosophical structure of psychiatry. *Am J Psych*. 2005; **162**: 433–40.
9 Lakoff G, Johnson M. *Metaphors We Live By*. Chicago, IL: University of Chicago Press; 1980.
10 Blasfield RK, Burgess DR. Classification provides an essential basis for organizing mental disorders. In: SO Lilienfeld, WT O'Donohue, editors. *The Great Ideas of Clinical Science*. New York: Routledge; 2007.
11 Zachar P. Psychiatric disorders are not natural kinds. *Philosophy, Psychiatry & Psychology*. 2001; 7: 167–82.
12 Gert B, Culver CM. Defining mental disorder. In: J Radden, editor. *Philosophy of Psychiatry. A Companion*. New York: Oxford University Press; 2004, pp. 414–25.
13 Wakefield JC. Disorder as harmful dysfunction: a conceptual critique of DSM-III-R's definition of mental disorder. *Psychological Review*. 1992; **99**: 232–47.
14 Lilienfeld SO, Marino L. Mental disorder as a Roschian concept: A critique of Wakefield's 'harmful dysfunction' analysis. *J Abnorm Psychol*. 1995; **104**: 411–20.
15 Megone C. Aristotle's function argument and the concept of mental illness. *Philosophy, Psychiatry & Psychology*. 1998; **5**: 187–201.
16 Ibid.
17 Sadler JZ. *Values and Psychiatric Diagnosis*. New York: Oxford University Press; 2005.
18 Ibid.
19 Sadler JZ. Diagnosis/antidiagnosis. In: J Radden, editor. *Philosophy of Psychiatry. A Companion*. New York: Oxford University Press; 2004, pp. 163–79.
20 Lakoff, Johnson, op. cit.

CHAPTER 10

Certainty

JOHN SAUNDERS

'Is there any knowledge in the world which is so certain that no reasonable man could doubt it? This question, which at first sight might not seem difficult, is really one of the most difficult that can be asked.' So begins Russell's *The Problems of Philosophy*.[1] From this beginning, Russell discusses the problems of appearance and reality. This question is fundamental to Western philosophy: what can I know? Or, perhaps more precisely, what can *I* know?

Descartes begins his *Discourse on Method* in a similar place. 'Of philosophy I will say nothing except that when I saw that it had been cultivated for many ages by the most distinguished men, and that yet there is not a single matter within its sphere which is not still in dispute, and nothing, therefore, which is above doubt.' Similarly, he begins his *Principles of Philosophy* by stating 'that in order to seek truth, it is necessary once in the course of our life to doubt, as far as possible, of all things . . . that we ought to consider as false all that is doubtful . . . that we ought not meanwhile to make use of doubt in the conduct of life.'[2]

Descartes goes on to assert that his ability to think is a demonstration of his existence and he is certain that he is not being deluded. Beyond his existence, however, he then raised the question whether he was deluded about the existence of his body and whether he might be a purely mental being. So doubt persisted and remained the starting point for his philosophy.

This may seem an odd place to start. For we are not concerned here with the metaphysical basis of knowledge. Doctors and patients do not doubt each other's existence. In our stories, Rachel does not truly think she is dreaming even if she rhetorically exclaims 'diabetic?' in seeming disbelief, nor does Geoff in his depressed or demented paralysis, appear to doubt the external reality of his internal experience. Nor even, in the main, do doctors or patients share doubts about the reality of the phenomena that have given rise to the consultation. The issue is rather, how doubtful is the diagnostic conclusion, how uncertain? And, following this, what does this mean for care of the patient, for my care?

At this level, while we may acknowledge the uncertainties of our existence in some theoretical way, we do believe that we know some things and that our knowing corresponds to an external reality (whatever theory of truth we sign up to). In acknowledging the demands of that reality, we make a commitment to both thought and action. We have doubts about aspects of that external reality. We are not sure whether the globe is warming, whether there will be a pandemic with massive mortality, whether the railways are stretched beyond capacity. But we can live with that. Of reality itself, there is no problem outside the saloon bar.

Diagnosis has often been taught as the supreme aspect of the doctor's art. Treatment of an active kind may be impossible, not available. But diagnosis remains important. Specialties like neurology formerly gloried in the ability to make diagnosis, but acknowledged that treatment was beyond its power. Diagnosis implied first the ability to name a symptom or collection of symptoms and signs. A label could be affixed. With the label came the assumption that the problem had been recognised. If not a 'disease', at least it might represent a syndrome – a collection of features whose association was known by someone, described in some paper or book and accepted through the social fabric of modern medicine. As discussed in the previous volume,[3] naming forces the experiential into the linguistic and enables us to begin understanding. Consider the following:

> The censorious game is an ancient medical tradition – some doctors are still uncertain whether they approve of sex – but the commonest version played today was shaped during the 1950s, with the coming of the hula hoop. Doctors discovered then that if they issued gloomy warnings about what hooping could do to the spine, not only did they get their letter into their professional journals but their names into the sort of newspapers read by their patients. They needed little further encouragement and recently, for instance, we've had grave pronouncements about Jogger's Nipple, Break-dancing Neck, Crab-eater's

Lung, Swim-goggle Headache, and Amusement Slide Anaphylaxis. Indeed, in the index of the New England Journal of Medicine, you can find Cyclist's Pudendum, Dog Walker's Elbow, Space Invaders' Wrist, Unicyclist's Sciatica, Jeans Folliculitis, Jogger's Kidney, Flautist's Neuropathy and Urban Cowboy's Rhabdomyolosis – a painful nastiness in the muscles caused by riding mechanical bucking broncos in amusement arcades.[4]

If we know the diagnosis – and know it with certainty – we can inform, act and prognosticate. No action can be confidently contemplated until we are prepared to make a commitment of sufficient strength to motivate change. Diagnostic uncertainty, at one level, is paralysing. For many doctors, there is even a reluctance to manage symptoms. As uncertainty diminishes so change follows: treatment perhaps, prognostication, more confident symptom control and, in the best practice, focussed empathy, understanding.

DIAGNOSTIC UNCERTAINTY AND UNDERSTANDING

Tennis elbow or housemaid's knee may not have the same ring as acute myelomonoblastic leukaemia or even the more commonplace diabetes, haemorrhoids, psoriasis, bronchial cancer and depression that our stories depict. But whatever the label, its importance has traditionally been the primary aim of the clinical encounter.

This act of labelling is profoundly important for patients as well as doctors. To carry the label gives a status. The processes and experiences have not only been named, but also recognised, somehow authorised. The sick role may have been legitimised, at least in most ordinary situations. But diagnosis goes beyond this. It also implies the determination of the nature of a diseased condition and in offering a diagnostic opinion, the doctor is also claiming an understanding of it. It makes sense, in that ordinary use of that word. The list of syndromes so amusingly set out in O'Donnell's writing has a more serious pedagogic value. The labels tell us something of the causes as well as providing identification. We understand the symptoms.

But even in more ordinary diagnostic boxes, what is diabetes or epilepsy? What is the boundary between non-diabetes or non-epilepsy and the real things? Certainty may be impossible about this; and given that the boundary conditions for such opinions may always be contested, the diagnosis may often be uncertain. What defines diabetes? For Rachel with her symptoms of drinking excessively and a need for insulin to remove such symptoms, the question seems absurd. But the diagnostic boundaries are as fluid as her literal symptoms. Here we have an example of a prognostic definition, based on something which is not of direct importance to either patient or doctor. For diabetes is defined as a disease characterised by a concentration of blood glucose that creates a risk of (asymptomatic) microaneurysms in the eye after an interval of time. The concentration is defined in a population that is unrepresentative of the majority that suffer the disease, varies according to the international authority that is consulted and the defining complication has been selected only because it creates a risk of something else, namely visual impairment. Diabetes at the boundary is, in truth, what others have said it is. We could cite other examples, such as hypertension, renal failure, chronic bronchitis or schizophrenia. Is one seizure enough to diagnose epilepsy? How many paranoid allegations or delusions or hallucinations to diagnose schizophrenia? How much cough or how high a blood pressure to diagnose chronic bronchitis or hypertension? Who says? And the answer is the magisterium of WHO or a learned national or international society.

Boundary conditions are often fluid, even for such seemingly 'hard' diagnoses as ischaemic heart disease. A myocardial infarct may be defined as a set of observations, in every case with a prescribed boundary. The boundary may be statistical, but that hardly gives it a clearly separated status from the normal. Indeed the overlap may be explicit. It is easily overlooked that normal ranges in many biochemical and other tests are defined as the mean plus or minus two standard deviations. The use of such statistical techniques to define a range for normally distributed data carries the implication that the top and bottom 2.5% will automatically be defined as abnormal. Many doctors still fail to think this through. The 2.5% false positive rate implies 25 false positives in every 1000 people randomly tested. For a disease with an incidence of 1 in a 1000 in the population, the chance of having the disease if the test is positive is therefore only 1 in 26. The test only becomes useful if the population has a much higher incidence – for which the usual test might be the appropriate clinical picture. Even then, a judgement will be needed as to the significance of the result – for which there can be no rule. Of course, how much uncertainty depends on the nature of the diagnosis. A diagnosis of viral disease may rest upon a clinical presentation and a rash that appears characteristic or it may rest upon a rise in titre of antibodies in the serum – the defining increase of which is itself another fluid boundary. A diagnosis of pulmonary embolism similarly may rest upon clinical judgement in an acute situation or a defined size of obstruction in a lung blood vessel on a scan.

Symptoms create their own challenges. When an abnormality is found on investigation, it is all too easy to assume that the symptom must be due to it – especially if the text books assure us that this is the case. An angiogram may show narrowing of the coronary blood vessels, but that is not sufficient to prove that the chest pain is due to coronary artery disease. An anatomical observation cannot, in this case, dictate a physiological conclusion. Or to take another example, malaise and exhaustion may result from hypercalcaemia, due in its turn to parathyroid disease. Equally, malaise and exhaustion are common in the general population and almost useless as screening symptoms. It is all too easy to ascribe the symptom to the hypercalcaemia if the latter is found on biochemical testing. These are the problems of misplaced inference in the diagnostic process – ascribing symptoms to diseases which may themselves be genuine on further investigation. Given the power of placebo treatment, it may always be uncertain how far the relationship is genuine in a given patient even after successful treatment – freedom from chest pain after a bypass graft or normalising blood calcium in these examples. Uncertainty will persist and the explanatory power of diagnosis will be diminished accordingly.

Does the disease exist at all? A court has expressed the opinion that Repetitive Strain Injury does not exist. The status of Gulf War Syndrome has been much debated and the existence of Chronic Fatigue Syndrome in children has been described in Britain, but apparently not in France. Here is a new slant on uncertainty in diagnosis: the cultural acceptance of certain labels,[5] especially where there are heated debates over psychosomatic mechanisms. But similar debates occur in more obviously physical 'conditions'. Is obesity a diagnosis? Or what certainty attaches itself to alcoholism (or is it just a description of an abusive behaviour)? Here our uncertainties seem to arise because of our attitudes to the conclusions that we reach. Obesity may create as much health risk as hypertension or hyperlipidaemia and certainly more than a solitary fit: but in general, we do not regard the fat person as diseased or even ill. Our categorisation of disease itself has its own uncertainties.

REDUCING UNCERTAINTIES

Whatever the irreducible core of uncertainty, both doctors and patients want as confident a diagnosis as possible, as well as a treatment recommendation that is as sure of providing maximum benefit as possible. Of course, there are routes to reducing such uncertainty. Diagnosis often proceeds in a hierarchy.

The process begins with the gathering of data, either by interviewing the patient or by taking an account from other witnesses or by observing the patient in his surroundings. Mostly, of course, it is the interview that is the key tool: an opportunity to establish a relationship, demonstrate concern, express empathy and collect data from a 'history'. The majority of diagnoses are established at this stage. Examination of the patient then enables those features to be found (or their absence established) that support the conclusion suggested by the history. Some patients require more than this: special investigations of some sort, such as blood tests or radiological imaging. As the process continues, uncertainty is usually reduced. For the conscious autonomous patient, the history is the single most important factor as well as the starting one, yet tests may be needed or even (unnecessarily) expected.

In an age that is fascinated by technology, patients and doctors have an almost mystical attachment to tests, lots of tests. The test may be almost worthless, but it often carries an air of greater certainty than any amount of wise bedside opinion. Moreover, the typed report of the X-ray, representing the opinion of one doctor trained to express an opinion about shadows, is viewed with awe, often ignoring the reality that certainty for that doctor too may not be possible. At the time of writing this chapter, I was caring for a patient whose isotope bone scan report confidently asserted that he had metastatic cancer in his skeleton. Therapists and junior doctors were eager to proceed on this basis, wishing to inform the patient of the finding. From a more experienced viewpoint, I was able to assert the improbability of such a conclusion and the conclusion of (probable) multiple osteoporotic fractures was made.

I also note an odd paradox here. Patients often want more tests when the outcomes are relatively trivial: CT scans for headaches that are confidently asserted by even a semi-competent doctor to be of no great importance – the perennial problem of the worried well, often generating still more anxiety as significant pathology is confused with normal variation. Yet the reduction of uncertainty when the diagnosis is of life-threatening importance becomes overwhelming. Even tests of doubtful or limited value may be pursued in, shall we say, possible motor neurone disease. Countless patients are offered electroencephalograms of doubtful value in an attempt to 'disprove' a diagnosis of epilepsy – an outcome that is logically impossible for an investigation that is, more often than not, normal even in *bona fide* cases.

As the diagnostic process continues, uncertainty is reduced. When it has been minimised, action may follow. Sometimes it doesn't work like this. Examination fails to support the conclusion confidently established or the investigations make it less likely. This is no seamless process to eradicate the uncertain.

Diagnosis may therefore have its first attraction as providing explanation. In psychiatry, that explanation may carry the added benefit of mitigation and exculpation in certain contexts. Diagnosis may also be reassuring. To know the problem is to have at least some prospect of coping with it – even the negative implications of so much traditional neurological diagnosis. There may be more sinister implications too. Diagnosis may transform social deviance into medical illness, especially in psychiatry. With this may come exclusion and dehumanisation. The roots of such thinking are widespread and primitive. Exclusion may lead to dehumanisation and the latter to conduct that would otherwise be unthinkable, especially in wartime.

For many doctors, guideline-based diagnosis helps to reduce uncertainty, or at least to reduce the feeling of uncertainty. Certain features of a disease may have been described in a certain percentage of patients, certain symptoms in another proportion and so the diagnosis is reached by some sort of scoring system. The diagnosis, as in the phrase that Dr Siddha (wrongly) uses of Jake, 'ticks all the boxes'. Such a process may help in a research context where categorising diagnoses into groups may be important in characterising a disorder. In some cases this gives rise to the debates around 'lumpers' and 'splitters': those who prefer to make a diagnosis of great precision and those who acknowledge the overlap of categories and prefer to lump all patients together. The splitters, for example, may prefer labels such as systemic lupus erythematosus or polyarteritis, the lumpers will be content with immunological connective tissue disease as a broader term. Alternatively, the guideline scoring system may aid a decision to proceed with treatment: this patient is said to have endocarditis after reaching a certain score and therefore to commence treatment for the next six weeks.

Part of the problem in this is the attempt to systematise the tacit. The experienced and reflective clinician will weigh clinical features in different ways. The same complaint will be given a different weight if coming from the stoical patient who never attends, rather than the patient who comes back every week; or in the patient whose complaint is expressed in a certain way or with other accompanying behavioural features. Bad pain is not easy to take seriously in a grinning patient. To the box ticker, all complaints are the same. Clinicians do, on occasions, sense the seriousness of a new complaint tacitly – one patient is taken more seriously for reasons that occasionally may be hard to express. The clinician may have detected the alarm in the voice, the hidden concern, the unusual word, yet may not be fully aware exactly what s/he is responding to. The guideline score is incapable of detecting this; it fails to systematise the tacit and could not do so even in principle. The ability to respond to these clues in diagnosis is not entirely dependent on explicit knowledge. A good clinician is not simply one who knows the text books better, but one who possesses a massive store of personal knowledge. It is the application of such personal knowledge that may enable the reduction in the diagnostic uncertainty.

The application of guideline medicine or of the algorithm provides a convenient prop for the inexperienced. The more expert know the shortcomings. But even allowing for the possibilities of computerising the decision tree and, at least, minimising the uncertainties arising from ignorance, the entry point remains crucial. Personal interaction involves the interpretation of language, a judgement that what was meant is what the listener thought was meant. Ambiguity or the habit of using words in different ways leads to different evaluations of meaning. The word 'flatulence', for example, even means different things to different doctors: to 19 of 40 gastroenterologists it meant passing wind upwards, to 7 passing wind through the rectum, and to 11 passing wind in either direction.[6] Other words such as 'pain' are even harder to interpret. 'Does the pain hurt?' is an odd question from one perspective, from another a necessary attempt to identify what is meant. Our vocabularies are the chief vehicles by which we express ourselves but, as discussed in Volume One, sometimes require a profound cultural understanding, especially in psychiatry or in the management of chronic disease.

The clinical algorithm originates from a method of computer programming known as flow chart construction. Flow charts mimic the Boolean logic that is built into digital computers and manipulates the logical operators *and*, *or*, and *not* in *if* statements. For example, *if* it is snowing *and* the fountains are turned off in Trafalgar Square *then* it is New Year's Eve.[7] Unfortunately the clinical realities are often more complex than the algorithm authors realise. Algorithms, like other approaches to diagnosis, may reduce uncertainty for the inexperienced, but the expert may be better placed to judge how uncertain is the conclusion.

Programmes of diagnostic logic aim to reduce uncertainty. They aim to enable a diagnosis to be reached based on a principle of parsimony, often using statistical theory to examine possibilities. The majority of work in the field of human judgement and decision making under uncertainty is based on the use and development of algebraic approaches, in which judgement is modelled in terms of mathematical choice functions. In the case of diagnosis, the most familiar approach has been the use of Bayes's theorem, an approach based on the prior probabilities of a given conclusion. This is a more economical approach than simply doing all the possible tests for a given symptom. Approaches of this sort can be modelled by computers and these may be more efficient than humans, especially at assessing the likelihood of the rare and recondite. Yet there is still a difficulty in selecting the entry point or in deciding whether a particular feature or symptom or sign counts. This is a personal judgement, which no computer could replace. 'The medical diagnostician's skill is as much an art of doing as it is an art of knowing . . . Connoisseurship, like skill, can be communicated only by example, not by precept . . . to be trained as a medical diagnostician, you must go through a long course of experience under the guidance of a master'[8] It is no use learning a list of syndromes in which the pulmonary component of the second heart sound may be accentuated: one must learn to recognise this sign in patients in whom it is authoritatively present compared to those in whom it is authoritatively absent. This art of knowing, asserts Polanyi, remains unspecifiable at the very heart of science. The relationship of pupil to master is that of an apprentice.

Others have tried to assert a process towards diagnosis that mimics the view of science described by Popper.[9] On this model the clinician makes a conjecture based on limited information and then tries to falsify it in further history, examination or investigation. In practice, however, clinicians are more likely to strive to verify a diagnosis as to falsify one.

Diagnostic logic and clinical decision making are virtually independent disciplines, with conceptual and practical considerations of great complexity, relating too to scientific studies of artificial intelligence. At present we may simply note that no explanation of human diagnostic logic so far conceived has been entirely satisfactory and no method of computer diagnosis has reduced diagnostic uncertainty to a degree sufficient for its widespread adoption.

SO WHAT IS CERTAIN DIAGNOSIS?

Dictionary definitions offer limited help, but provide a starting point for reflection: the determination of the nature of a diseased condition, identification of a disease by a careful investigation of its symptoms and history, also the opinion (formally stated) resulting from such investigation. The late Moran Campbell sets this out in more detail:

A disease is first recognised syndromally – a constellation of clinical features.

The disease has a cause (infective, nutritional, genetic, immunological etc.); this cause produces the characteristic structural changes, which in turn produce the clinical manifestations. The elucidation of the causative, structural and functional changes may not come in any particular historical order, but the paradigm has two characteristics: first, it is expected or at least hoped the relations will be specific (unique cause, unique structural and functional changes belonging to one syndrome). Second, as knowledge progresses, the defining process is 'pushed to the left' in the sequence given above. In other words, a disease will not be allowed to remain in syndromal terms if it can be explained or defined in functional terms; a functional syndrome will not be left in these terms if it can be characterised structurally, and 'cause' takes priority overall.[10]

Diagnostic certainty will only be achieved when the disease has been fully characterised. Rachel's diabetes, as presented to the reader, has not yet reached that diagnostic stage: we are not told and can only assume its cause. Jake's haemorrhoids may be related to long-standing constipation or to an undiagnosed bowel cancer: the account hardly opens up these possibilities; as for Geoff's depression, the reader has little idea of the disease in functional, let alone causal, terms. Uncertainty is greater than the casual reader may realise.

IF UNCERTAIN, IS IT IMPORTANT?

The question seems at first sight curious. Of course, diagnosis is important. The curse of so much medicine is the treating of symptoms without a clear understanding of mechanism of the sort described above by Campbell. Without a confident diagnosis, how can we advise Rachel of her treatment or Jen of her need for investigation or Jake of his need to adjust his diet? The strong emphasis on diagnosis seems obvious enough.

A counterexample may help, however. Suppose a patient has a blood pressure of 162/95 at the age of 69. Does it really matter whether we diagnose hypertension? What benefit for this patient is the label? There are no benefits to be claimed, no sick status, no time off work, no legitimation of any sick role. The diagnosis is not really important at all. The focus of interest is surely not: is the patient hypertensive? Rather the question is: what risk of stroke or cardiovascular complications does this patient run? Following from this comes the secondary question of what treatment should then be recommended. The emphasis is prognostic not diagnostic. Liz's not-yet-identified abnormal cells may come into just this category.

This is a circular argument and a tautologous one. For, surely, many diagnoses such as hypertension, diabetes and osteoporosis are defined on the basis of the risks they create of something else: stroke, blindness, hip fractures. The individual risk may demand no therapy, but the benefit for a significant proportion of the group with the appropriate characteristics is definitional. Certain diagnosis may not then be important for the individual in terms of individual treatment recommendations. But its importance cannot simply be denied and nothing more said.

Diagnosis may also have its importance for others. There may be little or no implication for an individual's treatment but a wider public interest. Supposing a patient has been exposed to an instrument such as an endoscope or a tonsillectomy knife used in a patient who was identified five years later as suffering from variant Creutzfeldt–Jacob disease. The risk to the individual who underwent the endoscopy or tonsillectomy may be calculated as, let us say, one in 75 at most. But there is a public health interest in minimising risk to others who might receive blood or organ transplants from the exposed patient. So this risk matters: if not chiefly or exclusively for the exposed patient, then for the public health. In advising on a diagnostic possibility with wide public health implications, minimising uncertainty becomes crucial.

Diagnostic uncertainty may also be important in the criminal justice system. Sally Clark was a solicitor who was convicted of killing her two children, who were found dead in their cots. The conviction was upheld on first appeal, only to be deemed unsafe on second appeal when it was discovered that certain test results had not been revealed to the court by an expert witness. But the declaration of Mrs Clark's innocence still left the diagnostic question open. What was the diagnosis causing the death of these children? It remains unanswered with any certainty, despite lengthy debate.[11] Such diagnostic dilemmas are well known in analysing cot deaths, especially where it may occur twice in one family.

Diagnosis matters. Reducing its uncertainty matters.

DIAGNOSTIC UNCERTAINTY AND EVIDENCE

Better knowledge helps to reduce uncertainty. Where there is uncertainty in knowledge, properly designed studies will reduce its extent. Many patients have difficulty in understanding uncertainty in medicine. Even in this day and age there is a quaint, yet widespread belief that doctors know what is happening. Hence, patients often find it hard to understand the rationale for clinical trials or studies of any sort. Why do it? Surely the doctor knows best.

The accumulation and validation of evidence lies at the heart of the evidence-based medicine movement (EBM). The practice of evidence-based medicine has changed the role of the physician from information dispenser to gatherer and analyser. The question that EBM attempts to answer is: what should we do if, after due reflection and consideration, we are uncertain of the diagnosis? To which the answer is that we must seek more evidence through a variety of studies that will reduce our areas of ignorance and our uncertainties. If we do not know what our strategy should be in achieving a diagnosis, then we should study situations systematically to achieve a more economical and more accurate strategy. Should Jake proceed to colonoscopy? What is the best way forward for the further investigation of Jen's chest complaints? If these strategies are uncertain, then better studies should inform our policies. Dr Siddha offers a menu, not information – and even that information is hardly accurate. Colonoscopy is trivialised by the phrase 'nothing too invasive' (Dr Siddha has obviously never experienced it), and irritable bowel syndrome isn't characterised by haemorrhoids (perhaps Dr Siddha needs a revision course).

Whatever its history, the EBM movement remains our most reliable tool for reducing uncertainty in diagnosis, in investigational strategies and in treatment too; our best hope of designing a map to traverse the grey zones of medicine. But at its heart lies its epidemiological nature. That is the nature of the evidence if offers: based on studies not of one but of a population of patients. Herein lies its weakness also. For the application of generalisations established by the study of populations to individuals creates a problem. The benefits of EBM may be statistically sound, the study design impeccable, but within the population studied there may be much variation. Some may benefit less than others, some may even be harmed even if overall there is a general benefit. The diagnostic strategy that results may not apply to all. This difficulty is incorrigible and no amount of statistical jiggery-pokery can avoid it.[12] The personal judgements of the doctor remain crucial in applying EBM to this patient, of this age, with these co-morbidities, in this situation. Even EBM cannot remove diagnostic uncertainty.

The typical 'evidence-based' review identifies a large number of articles and then discards many as irrelevant and many more as methodologically unsound. The review is then based on the remaining handful and by implication all the other articles have nothing to contribute. However, detailed knowledge of the subject is often needed to judge the worth of a paper, and even methodologically flawed articles often contribute some information to the evidence base. In addition, errors in peer review occur; researchers can be biased; numbers are misrepresented to prove hypotheses, and the structure of the study may be misrepresentative of underlying truths concerning the results, such as characteristics of the subjects or length of the study.

Nearly always other information and judgement are required to interpret the general conclusions of EBM. The wise clinician will consider all the information, formalised and informal, available before making a decision. As one commentator has said, in an uncertain world, judgement-free medicine is as bad or worse than evidence-free.[13]

The extent of these judgements often surprise the naïve. Firstly, judgement is exercised in deciding what data to collect in establishing the corpus of evidence-based medicine. Faced with the patient, a similar judgement is made in deciding on a particular line of inquiry. No doctor faces the patient with no idea on the direction of inquiry. Sometimes this may be quite detailed. Faced with a fat, forty-year-old female with abdominal pain, there may be an early focus on the gall bladder; while a patient with, shall we say, the typical facial appearance of acromegaly or Cushing's syndrome will have the inquiry focussed on those possibilities before even speaking. Judgement, too, will be exercised in the interpretation of the history, especially in diagnoses where no further confirmation is possible. Migraine or trigeminal neuralgia are specific syndromes with specific treatments and there is a need for the greatest possible certainty in diagnosis to inform therapy. Both will depend on a judgement on the story, a decision as to how far the features represent the typical pictures described in the medical literature. Similarly, judgement may be exercised in examination: is this reflex pathologically brisk, is this optic disc actually swollen? No computer can do this. And finally, in the investigative process judgement is needed again: is this biopsy composed of malignant tissue or is this appearance on X-ray outside the normal and therefore significant? These judgements require a huge experience for which there is no substitute. They also require the personal qualities to have reflected on and learnt from that experience. No text book or course can replace the personal knowledge of such a practitioner.

These themes have been explored in Polanyi's concept of personal knowledge.[14] In scientific discovery, personal judgement is brought to bear in a way that cannot be described even in principle. There is an element of connoisseurship in arriving at such judgements, just as there is in identifying (diagnosing?) a fine wine, portraying a Shakespearian character or making a Stradivarius violin. The roots for such knowing may be mainly tacit and no computer could replace them.

EXPRESSING DIAGNOSTIC UNCERTAINTY AND ITS EFFECTS

It is suggested that doctors should be more open in expressing uncertainty, whether in diagnosis or treatment or prognosis. The days are long past when patients passively accept what is said and the doctor-patient relationship is surely healthier for that. In reality we know that informed decision making is often lacking, especially in complex decisions. Assessment of patient understanding of uncertainty is particularly problematic and rarely adequately performed. In the past, some have argued that doctors are trained to display an air of confidence and ignore uncertainties or that they are trained to accept them uncritically. Perhaps uncertainties are even to be desired. For a total elimination of uncertainty would lead to a deterministic life, meaning that all events would be known in advance, in turn implying no hope, no ethics, no freedom of choice. Perhaps too disclosure of uncertainty will have a negative effect on patient confidence, trust, satisfaction and hope.[15] One study showed a strong correlation between disclosing uncertainty and increased patient dissatisfaction. It may be however be that the way and the time are the more critical factors in the act of the disclosure.

However, by disclosing uncertainties the doctor contributes potentially vital information for the patient's decision making. The patient is better informed and patient autonomy is enhanced. Concerns that would otherwise be hidden can be addressed and there will be a significant impact on understanding. Using appropriate skills, the result should be shared decision making and a better understanding of the judgements behind the doctor's recommendations. As disclosure of uncertainty becomes commonplace in medical practice, the doctor/patient relationship will evolve to a level of greater understanding and satisfaction for both the doctor and patient.

Disclosure creates its ethical challenges. How strong should a diagnostic anxiety be for disclosure? A diabetic patient walks into the clinic and is noticed to have muscle fasciculations. They have been present for 10 years and he has additional muscle wasting in an arm and one leg. His symptoms are entirely additional to those that have led to the consultation and appear to have no connection. What should be said? The untreatable fatal disease of motor neurone disease presents with muscle wasting and fasciculation, but 10 years is unusual. Is this possible? Nothing is said beyond the need to investigate further. A nerve conduction velocity study is arranged and the conclusion is one of probable diabetic neuropathy. The patient has been spared the disturbing possibilities that have arisen from the doctor's uncertainties. To share all one's thoughts may be the demand of a thoroughgoing openness, but few will find the time or the courage to be so frank; and most patients may not benefit as a result. Sometimes uncertainty must be the doctor's secret rather than abandoning the patient to his or her uncertainties. Expression of uncertainty may be verbal or behavioural. A doctor may say that he doesn't know or is uncertain of the diagnosis; or he may scratch his head, furrow his brow, avoid saying anything at all or simply obfuscate ('we'll do some tests'). Rachel's doctor smiles, Jake's talks as if it's all everyday and continues writing as she speaks. All the doctors in our stories seem to be in the reassurance business.

The actions taken may have a different impact on the patients. For example, an expression of uncertainty such as 'Let's see what happens' was perceived as potentially damaging to patient confidence in a survey of both patients and doctors.[16] Perhaps surprisingly, in the same study both patients and doctors found that asking a nurse for advice would also have a detrimental effect. On the other hand, a behaviour such as looking something up in a book or doing a search on the computer was viewed more positively. Patients were far less troubled by the effect of verbal expressions of uncertainty on their confidence than doctors. These reactions were found to depend on certain characteristics in the patient. Those of lower social class (probably less well educated), those younger and those who had known their doctor for a shorter period had the greatest negative response to any expression of uncertainty.

IS THE BEST DOCTOR UNCERTAIN?

Increasing use of diagnostic technologies – laboratory tests, imaging procedures, electrophysiological investigations etc. – may decrease some uncertainties but increase others. New diagnostic possibilities create new room for doubt. The more we know, the more we realise we have to find out. Our uncertainties may increase. Campbell's move to the left becomes harder to make.

The more perceptive doctor may be the one who is the more uncertain. Only the ignorant believe that knowledge is finite and capable of being boxed away in an unalterable category. An intimation of fruitfulness is the sign of the most significant discoveries. A fruitful discovery leads to new truths. Of course, fruitfulness itself cannot be a criterion of truth for the implications of any new discovery, be it scientific law or diagnosis, cannot always be known immediately. In science, at the time we have made up our minds about the merits of a discovery, its future repercussions are still unknown. You cannot, as the Bellman advised, spot a Snark by its habit of dining the following day.[17] Fruitfulness appears as an intimation of future realities. A diagnosis of epilepsy rather than syncope is not true because its implications are more far reaching. But a true diagnosis is more fruitful for the life of the patient than a wrong one in a potentially huge number of ways.

Philosophy, according to Descartes, had to start afresh by ridding itself of all preconceptions, however indispensable they seemed. Radical doubt was Descartes' starting place and from it he reconstructed a view of reality that he held to be true. In so doing, new insights into the philosophical world view were attained. It would be fanciful to see such ambitions in a radical scepticism about diagnosis. But certainly on occasions, the doctor has to sit back, return to basic observations and attempt a reconstruction of the patient's problem and its explanation. The best diagnostician is more than Osler's aphorism as one with one finger down the throat and one in the rectum, although the emphasis on clinical skills is real enough.

'If you dissemble sometimes your knowledge of that you are thought to know, you shall be thought, another time, to know that which you know not,' wrote Francis Bacon.[18] But the doctors' days of dissembling are long over. No-one need regret their passing.

REFERENCES

1 Russell B. *The Problems of Philosophy*. London: Thornton Butterworth; 1912.
2 Descartes R. *A Discourse on Method*, trans. J Veitch. London: JM Dent; 1912.
3 Saunders J. Vocabulary of health and illness. In: M Evans, R Ahlzén, I Heath, J Macnaughton, editors. *Medical Humanities Companion. Volume 1 Symptom*. Oxford: Radcliffe Publishing; 2008, p. 64.
4 O'Donnell M. *Doctor, Doctor: an insider's guide to the games doctors play*. London: Orion; 1986.
5 Clare A. National variations in medical practice. *BMJ*. 1989; **298**: 1334.
6 Knill-Jones R. A formal approach to symptoms in dyspepsia. *Clin Gastroenterol*. 1985; **14**: 517–19.
7 Macartney F. Diagnostic logic. In: C Phillips. *Logic in Medicine*. British Medical Journal: London; 1988, pp. 33–58.
8 Polanyi M. *Personal Knowledge*. London: Routledge & Kegan Paul; 1958, p. 54.
9 Popper K. *Logic der Forschung*. Berlin: Springer; 1934.
10 Campbell A. The science of diagnosis. In: C Phillips, J Wolfe, editors. *Clinical Practice and Economics*. London: Pitman Publishing; 1977, pp. 101–12.
11 Horton R. In defence of Roy Meadow. *Lancet*. 2005; **366**: 3–5.
12 Charlton B. Book review of evidence-based medicine. *J Eval Clin Pract*. 1997; **3**: 169–72.
13 Kemm J. Well informed uncertainties about the effects of treatment: 'Evidence based' must not equal 'judgment free'. *BMJ*. 2004; **328**: 1018.
14 Polanyi M, op. cit.

15 Parascandola M, Hawkins J, Danis M. Patient autonomy and the challenge of clinical uncertainty. *Kennedy Inst Ethics J.* 2002; **12**: 245–64.

16 *Patient Education and Counselling.* 2002; **48**: 171–6.

17 Carroll L. The hunting of the Snark (Fit the second). In: J Cohen, editor. *More Comic & Curious Verse*. Harmondsworth: Penguin Books; 1956, pp. 103–23. A famous English nonsense poem:

> Come, listen my men, while I tell you again
> The five unmistakable marks
> By which you may know, wheresoever you go,
> The warranted genuine Snarks.
> Its habit of getting up late you'll agree
> That it carries too far, when I say
> That it frequently breakfasts at five o'clock tea,
> And dines on the following day.

18 Bacon F. Of discourse. *Essays XXXII* (1597). London: Dent; 1906.

Index